Academy of Nutrition and Dietetics

POCKET GUIDE TO

Eating Disorders

THIRD EDITION

Jessica Setnick
MS, RD, CEDS-C

Academy of Nutrition and Dietetics
Chicago, IL

Academy of Nutrition and Dietetics

Academy of Nutrition and Dietetics
120 S. Riverside Plaza, Suite 2190
Chicago, IL 60606

Academy of Nutrition and Dietetics Pocket Guide to Eating Disorders, Third Edition

ISBN 978-0-88091-236-5 (print)
ISBN 978-0-88091-237-2 (eBook)
Catalog Number 436X25 (print)
Catalog Number 436X25e (eBook)

The views expressed in this publication are those of the authors and do not necessarily reflect policies and/or official positions of the Academy of Nutrition and Dietetics. Mention of product names in this publication does not constitute endorsement by the authors or the Academy of Nutrition and Dietetics. The Academy of Nutrition and Dietetics disclaims responsibility for the application of the information contained herein.

10 9 8 7 6 5 4 3 2 1

For more information on the Academy of Nutrition and Dietetics, visit www.eatright.org.

Library of Congress Cataloging-in-Publication Data

Names: Setnick, Jessica, author.
Title: Pocket guide to eating disorders / Jessica Setnick, MS, RD, CEDS-C.
Other titles: Eating disorders
Description: Third edition. | Chicago, IL : Academy of Nutrition and Dietetics, 2025. | Includes bibliographical references and index.
Identifiers: LCCN 2024059090 (print) | LCCN 2024059091 (ebook) | ISBN 9780880912365 (spiral bound) | ISBN 9780880912372 (ebook)
Subjects: LCSH: Eating disorders--Diet therapy--Handbooks, manuals, etc.
Classification: LCC RC552.E18 S48 2025 (print) | LCC RC552.E18 (ebook) | DDC 616.85/260654--dc23/eng/20250218
LC record available at https://lccn.loc.gov/2024059090
LC ebook record available at https://lccn.loc.gov/2024059091

Contents

Contents

List of Boxes, Tables, and Figures

Boxes

Table

Figure

Frequently Used Terms and Abbreviations

ACT	acceptance and commitment therapy
ADHD	attention-deficit with hyperactivity disorder
AN	anorexia nervosa
APA	American Psychiatric Association
ARFID	avoidant/restrictive food intake disorder
BED	binge-eating disorder
BN	bulimia nervosa
CBT	cognitive behavioral therapy
CFS	chronic fatigue syndrome
DBT	dialectical behavior therapy
DEB	Dysfunctional Eating Behavior
DEXA/DXA	dual-energy x-ray absorptiometry scan
DSM-5-TR	*Diagnostic and Statistical Manual of Mental Disorders, 5th Edition, Text Revision*
ED	eating disorder
EFFT	emotion-focused family therapy
EKG/ECG	electrocardiogram

EMDR	eye movement desensitization and reprocessing
FBT	family-based treatment
FDA	US Food and Drug Administration
ICD-10-CM	*International Classification of Diseases*, 10th Revision, Clinical Modification
IFEDD	International Federation of Eating Disorder Dietitians
IFS	internal family systems
MHPAEA	Mental Health Parity and Addiction Equity Act of 2008
MI	motivational interviewing
MNT	medical nutrition therapy
NCP	Nutrition Care Process
NES	night eating syndrome
NFPE	nutrition focused physical examination
OCD	obsessive-compulsive disorder
ON	orthorexia nervosa
ONS	oral nutrition supplements
OSFED	other specified feeding and eating disorders
PCOS	polycystic ovary syndrome
PD	purging disorder
PES	problem, etiology, signs/symptoms
PN	parenteral nutrition
PTSD	post-traumatic stress disorder
RD	rumination disorder
RDN	registered dietitian nutritionist
REDs	relative energy deficiency in sport
SE	somatic experiencing
WHO	World Health Organization

Reviewers

Quinn Haisley, MS, RD
Owner and Registered Dietitian, Practice Eros Nutrition
Astoria, NY

Kimmie Singh, MS, RD, CDN
Registered Dietitian, Body Honor Nutrition
New York, NY

Brianna Theus, RD
Registered Dietitian, The Celestial Life
Shelton, CT

Preface and Acknowledgments

Welcome to the third edition of the *Academy of Nutrition and Dietetics Pocket Guide to Eating Disorders*. My goal with the first two editions was to equip dietitians with concise, accessible, and evidence-based information to guide practice and improve outcomes for individuals with eating disorders. With this edition I added a new goal: to create a fully inclusive depiction of eating disorders that finally lays to rest the outdated and harmful stereotypes that have long permeated our field. I am grateful to the reviewers, Brianna Theus, RD; Quinn Haisley, MS, RD; and Kimmie Singh, MS, RD, CDN, for helping me meet that challenge.

This book would never have made it into your hands or onto your screen without my amazingly patient and dedicated editor Stacey Zettle, MS, RDN; Betsy Hornick, MS, RDN; and everyone on the Academy of Nutrition and Dietetics production team working behind the scenes. We all hope this new edition of *Pocket Guide to Eating Disorders* will serve as a valuable resource in your work.

Finally, allow me to thank you for all you're doing to ensure a better future for your patients. Your dedication to supporting individuals through their recovery is the reason this book exists.

With gratitude,

Jessica Setnick, MS, RD, CEDS-C

About the Author

Jessica Setnick, MS, RD, CEDS-C, is known to dietitians worldwide as an expert in eating disorder nutrition counseling. For the past 26 years, she has worked in every level of eating disorder care and education as a dietitian, speaker, and consultant. Her signature training workshop for health professionals, Eating Disorders Boot Camp, has been attended by thousands of dietitians and other professionals since 2003. She is the author of *The Academy of Nutrition and Dietetics Pocket Guide to Eating Disorders* and several other books.

In 2012, Jessica founded the International Federation of Eating Disorder Dietitians (IFEDD), which has grown to nearly 1,000 members worldwide. Through IFEDD and the Access to Care Project, Jessica advocates to expand access to eating disorder care and against insurance company discrimination and harmful stereotypes.

In 2019, Jessica shared insights into her decades of public speaking experience in *A Dietitian's Guide to Professional Speaking: Expert Advice for Pitching, Presenting & Getting Paid!*, and most recently starting touring the country again with her workshop Healing Your Inner Eater. Jessica's passion is supporting dietitians, so after decades of advising other RDNs, she put all of the most common questions into *The Sleepless Dietitian's Guide: Advice for the Angst That Keeps You Up at Night*. She envisions a world where no one is ashamed to talk about their eating issues and anyone who wants help can get it. Contact Jessica at Jessica@UnderstandingNutrition.com or visit www.JessicaSetnick.com.

CHAPTER 1

Eating Disorders and the Dietitian

"How innocent we were when we thought working with eating disorders was a choice."

-Sherry Tarleton, RDN, CNSC

Introduction

Every registered dietitian nutritionist (RDN) needs a working knowledge of eating disorders. It doesn't matter if eating disorders are not your specific practice area; you will encounter individuals with dysfunctional eating behaviors anywhere you work with other humans. Eating disorders are a part of every general and specialty nutrition practice, population, and group because they can affect anyone who eats. And for the most part, the effects are negative. Although sometimes initiated because they seem helpful, when pursued to extremes, eating disorders can cause disease, disability, death, and incredible physical and mental suffering.

Contrary to how it may appear at first glance, the eating disorder field is a work in progress. Causes of eating disorders are still largely unknown. Research on methods of treatment is in its infancy and riddled with controversies. There is no one agreed-upon treatment and no consensus definition of recovery. Topics such as end-of-life care, family participation, and whether eating disorders can be cured are still open to debate.

RDNs who specialize in eating disorders have for the most part remained above the fray by focusing on patient-centered, individualized medical nutrition therapy using the Nutrition Care Process. We adapt what we offer to each person, knowing that each of them—and their nutrition—will continue to change throughout their life. We follow the ethical standards of our profession: autonomy, beneficence, and justice.[1] This is nonnegotiable and does not rely on a person having been diagnosed with an eating disorder or even being willing to accept such a diagnosis.

The RDN stance is simple: all individuals experiencing eating disorders deserve access to compassionate assessment, recommendations for rehabilitative nutrition, and assistance with implementation. Our ultimate goals reflect our hope for each person to reach their full potential, even as we accept that these goals are not always attainable. They include:

- medical, psychological, and physical safety and health, free from weight bias;
- adequate nourishment, with dignity and without fear;
- enjoyable and safe movement, whether independently or in a community, in accordance with ability and preference ;
- autonomy to experience or refrain from new foods and freedom from food guilt; and
- body respect, from themselves and others, including comfortable clothes and accommodations, and respect for gender identity.

And even as we hope for these outcomes, we acknowledge the roles of systemic injustices and historic inequities that no amount of individual responsibility can overcome.

According to a comprehensive report published in 2020, 21 million US residents currently have eating disorders and, based on current patterns, 7.8 million more will develop an eating disorder in their lifetimes.[2] There is a shocking lack of awareness among public health, medical, and even mental health advocacy organizations about how prevalent eating disorders are, leading to indefensible disparities in research and research funds compared with other conditions.[3] Only a small fraction of individuals with eating disorders are ever diagnosed, and an even smaller number enter, much less complete, specialty treatment.[4-6] Even deaths from eating disorders are likely under-reported, as they are often attributed to suicide or heart failure, and the US Centers for Disease Control and Prevention do not track eating disorders as a cause of death.

The most significant driver of these problems is a gross misunderstanding of this basic fact: *anyone who eats can have an eating disorder*. Public perception, health care providers, and even eating disorder researchers remain mistaken about who develops eating disorders, what "counts" as an eating disorder, and how a person with an eating disorder looks. These biases are woven into the fabric of eating disorder treatment because of its basis in academic research during a period when anorexia nervosa was the only identified eating disorder and was believed to only affect females. Treatment strategies, recovery rates, and even diagnostic criteria were all based on the "SWAG" stereotype—shorthand for skinny, White, affluent (or adolescent) girl, even though most people with eating disorders do not meet that description.

Thankfully, finally, belatedly, research on eating disorder prevalence in the real world, among all types of people, has begun to be published, bringing awareness to what RDNs in the field have known all along—eating disorders do not discriminate. Individuals with eating disorders are at least as likely to identify as Black, Indigenous, Asian, Latine, or biracial and to be fat, transgender, poor, elderly, pregnant, in foster care, incarcerated, serving or previously having served in the military, on Medicaid, or more than one of these.[5-16] But because these groups have been historically excluded from eating disorder research and care, their members are less likely to be diagnosed with eating disorders, and therefore very unlikely to get specialty eating disorder care.

Moving forward, better education for medical and mental health professionals, more widespread information for the public, targeted research, and a wider variety of treatment options for eating disorders are needed. This will ensure that a) no eating disorder is missed due to ignorance, b) everyone who wants care for their eating disorder can access it, and c) that eating disorder care is beneficial and not stigmatizing, uninformed, or harmful.

The Dietitian's Role

Because we are skillful observers of the diverse range of human eating behaviors, RDNs are often the first to notice eating-related problems, whether among patients, students, colleagues, family members, or friends. Many of us were motivated to pursue nutrition as a career because of past experiences with our own or a loved one's eating disorder.[17-19] But the general dietetics education path rarely provides adequate skills to address the issues we find in practice.[20-23] Some forward-thinking educators and internship directors include eating disorders in their curricula beyond the very limited requirements, but the majority of RDNs are left to our own devices to find the information we need. In the years when the Academy of Nutrition and Dietetics Food & Nutrition Conference & Expo (FNCE®) includes eating disorder topics, these sessions are very well attended. Other times, eating disorders seem to be excluded from the larger conversation about nutrition and dietetics.

RDNs may be the first to identify problematic eating behaviors simply because we're looking deeply into each patient's nutrition. Once educated beyond the stereotypes, RDNs can be open to the many faces of eating disorders and the many ways they hide. We ask the questions no one else has asked, and we're excellent at sifting through information to find the facts, as well as what may remain unspoken. We can be good listeners who don't pass judgment or shame people for their eating behaviors. This allows our patients to share things they have never confided in anyone else. We offer building blocks for nutritional rehabilitation for individuals and education for the community. We raise awareness of the factors known to cause eating disorders and of their early warning symptoms. When given the opportunity, we can identify eating disorders at their earliest stages and ultimately we can change the course of lives.

Box 1.1 lists some of the many functions an RDN may play in the treatment of eating disorders. Box 1.2 on page 7 lists the outcomes of RDN nutrition counseling from the patient's point of view.

In addition to our important roles identifying and promoting healing from eating disorders, RDNs are leaders in the wider eating disorder field.[20,24,25] We lead clinical teams, we lead community organizations, and

BOX 1.1 Sample Roles of a Dietitian in the Treatment of Eating Disorders

Evaluate the patient's current eating patterns and identify their stated needs and goals.

Share findings and recommendations with the patient and other members of the medical and mental health teams.

Explain the role of nutrition and eating in physical and mental well-being and provide education to challenge inaccurate beliefs about food, while considering social determinants of health and respecting personal and cultural preferences.

Help the patient determine how to implement needed nutritional recommendations within the context of their abilities, level of family or community support, access to food, cultural heritage and experiences, and address difficulties with implementation.

Help the patient create an action plan with agreed-upon steps to repair nutritional deficiencies and work toward their goals. Follow up on action plans and modify as more information is received.

Identify nutrition knowledge and skill deficits. Assist the patient in gaining needed information and skills.

Offer active learning activities when appropriate, such as cooking, eating, and online or in-person grocery shopping, to help teach new behaviors and acceptance of food-related tasks and environments. Model appropriate eating in shared experiential interventions such as restaurant meals.

Educate about the harms of detrimental comments and beliefs around food, eating, and body size. Identify which of these may respond to intervention vs those which are not within the patient's control. Address these when within the registered dietitian's scope of practice and refer to other providers as needed.

Assist the patient in recognizing the impact of weight stigma, diet culture, and social determinants of health in their life and present options for managing them (when possible) in medical, social, and other settings.

Include other members of the interdisciplinary treatment team, family members, significant others, support partners, and so on, in sessions as appropriate; educate regarding eating disorders and nutrition as they relate to the patient's treatment plan and recovery needs.

Refer to additional care as needed, including specialty medical care, psychiatry, mental health care, and other treatment levels.

Continued on next page

BOX 1.1 Sample Roles of a Dietitian in the Treatment of Eating Disorders (cont.)

Teach group nutrition classes to patients, their families, and support partners, and lead group nutrition discussions that allow participants to express their thoughts and feelings, provide and receive support, address their experiences of diet culture and dysfunctional eating, and promote improved nutrition.

Document, publish, and share experiences, research findings, and outcomes to advance the field.

we lead by example. RDNs working in this area bridge medical and mental health, develop treatment programs and protocols, educate, counsel, supervise, and convey crucial information to other disciplines.[24] Considering that fewer than one in 10 medical residencies require an eating disorder rotation,[26] the RDN often has the most eating disorder expertise among a patient's health care providers.

RDNs contribute to advances in eating disorder treatment at every level of care.[21,24,25] We've practiced strategies such as harm avoidance, weight inclusivity, and family involvement long before they had names or became buzzwords in the field. Eating disorder professional organizations and advocacy groups with position statements all recognize medical nutrition therapy from an RDN to be a standard pillar of eating disorder care. Why then do some eating disorder treatment methodologies or professionals overlook the RDN's role in eating disorder treatment? Because they limit their search to scientific journals in their own field. Although RDNs have written hundreds of books and articles about our work, these are essentially invisible to researchers from other professions who rely only on what is published in peer-reviewed journals. Combined with the common practice of folding an RDN's contribution to patient care into the general umbrella of "treatment as usual," the relative scarcity of RDNs publishing about eating disorders in peer-reviewed journals is a major barrier to recognition of our role.

A significant roadblock to publishing in journals is that these types of publications require that all research must be approved in advance by an Institutional Review Board (IRB). For decades, only RDNs affiliated

BOX 1.2 Sample Outcomes of Dietitian-Led Nutrition Counseling

Improved ability to obtain and prepare food
Improved eating frequency or timing
Improved ability to plan for eating opportunities
Improved food, energy, and nutrient intake
Increased variety of foods
Increased comfort with trying unfamiliar foods
Increased comfort with social eating opportunities
Decreased preoccupation with food
Decreased compensatory behaviors after eating
Decreased shame about eating
Decreased loss-of-control eating episodes
Increased comfort or better boundaries around food and eating-related topics and questions
Improved understanding and acceptance of feelings about food
Improved ability to separate food and feelings and manage both appropriately
Improved ability to detect and follow internal hunger and satiety cues
Improved understanding of body weight and size changes over time
Improved understanding of body image and influences on body image
Increased understanding of weight stigma and tools to use when encountering it
Decreased punitive or excessive weight or body checking
Improved understanding of the process of eating disorder recovery

Adapted with permission from reference 20: Setnick J. Interventions used in nutrition counseling for eating disorder treatment: survey results. *SCAN's Pulse*. 2012;31(3).

with a large institution such as a hospital or university had access to an IRB. This roadblock was removed in 2023, when the International Federation of Eating Disorder Dietitians (IFEDD) established an IRB for use by RDNs. Increased published research on what RDNs contribute to the eating disorder field is crucial to increasing insurance coverage, research funding, and understanding of our essential role.

Future RDN training should include more awareness of eating disorders and prepare us to take leadership roles in the wider eating disorder field, in eating disorder research, and in eating disorder treatment settings. Our field must also welcome—and recruit!—many more dietitians who are Black, Indigenous, Asian, Pacific Islander, Latine, multiracial, fat, gender diverse, first-generation American, disabled, neurodivergent, and every other identity that our patients share. Eating disorder treatment can and will be better when more voices and experiences are included.

Am I Ready?

Every RDN has something to offer an individual experiencing an eating disorder. The primary requirements are authentic curiosity, respect for autonomy, and willingness to seek guidance from a more experienced RDN when needed. As a specialty practice area, working with individuals experiencing eating disorders can be intense and draining, and to be most effective, requires additional training beyond what is provided in school and internship programs.[21,24,27,28]

If you're new to eating disorder care, do not try to go it alone. Reach out to your supervisor, mental health professionals at your workplace, a networking group for eating disorder professionals such as IFEDD, or a more experienced RDN for guidance. Consider asking your workplace to pay for consultation sessions with an eating disorder specialist dietitian (often referred to as "professional supervision") for assistance with the personal aspects of working in eating disorder care as well as case consultation. When selecting continuing education, focus on eating disorders as well as counseling and mental health topics.

If you find yourself doubting your patient care decisions or thinking about work after hours, know that these are common reactions, not signs that you are making mistakes. Try not to feel embarrassed if you don't know something. The eating disorders field is filled with controversies and unanswered questions, and even experts do not have all the answers. Your best assets are curiosity and a willingness to reach out for support.

If you realize you're not interested in the field, you're not sympathetic toward individuals with eating disorders, or you're easily frustrated with slow or little progress, you may choose a different area of practice. When you encounter an individual with an eating disorder, as you occasionally will regardless of your specialty, speak with your supervisor for guidance and refer the individual to a different RDN if possible.

Even with an affinity for eating disorder treatment, you will encounter individuals whose needs exceed what you can provide. When you feel overwhelmed, get support from your own mental health provider or therapist, your professional supervisor/consultant, or peers. Finally, but importantly, if you're experiencing an eating disorder or you notice unhealthy thoughts or behaviors after a long day of helping others with eating disorders, know that this does not disqualify you from work as an RDN. You do need to seek help, and you may choose not to work with this patient population for a period of time. To be able to care for both your patients and yourself, you need awareness of your own thoughts, stressors, and behaviors as well as active engagement in your own recovery. This assures that when you're with patients, you can meet their needs without disregarding your own, and you can keep your own eating issues separate from the needs of your patients. A meeting with an experienced mental health professional or RDN is a starting place to assess your own relationship with food and determine how to proceed.

The Nutrition Care Process

This book is intended to prepare you for when you encounter an individual with an eating disorder in your professional life. The Nutrition Care Process format is followed throughout the remaining chapters. The Nutrition Care Process is comprised of four steps (assessment, diagnosis, intervention, and monitoring/evaluation) and is outlined in detail in Appendix A on page 169.

A Note on Terminology Used Throughout This Book

The following list details specific terminology used throughout the remainder of this book.

- "Dysfunctional eating behaviors" is used as an umbrella term for all eating and food-related activities that detract from an individual's nutritional health, regardless of the presence or absence of a formal eating disorder diagnosis
- "Patient" is used as a general term for someone experiencing an eating disorder and is interchangeable with "client" or "individual."
- "Support partners" is used to denote the wide range of individuals who may be participating in an individual's care, including caregivers, family members, parents, foster parents, siblings, spouses, significant others, children, legal guardians, home health care workers, family of choice, and others.
- "Supervisor" is used to describe a more experienced professional that an RDN can consult with about challenging situations, and can be someone such as a workplace supervisor, a paid consultant, or mentor.
- "Remote health care delivery" is used to describe phone, video, or online consultations and monitoring and is synonymous with "virtual health care" and "telemedicine."
- "Fat" is used as a neutral descriptor of body size as used by the fat-activist community.

References

1. Academy of Nutrition and Dietetics, Commission on Dietetic Registration. Code of Ethics for the Nutrition and Dietetics Profession. June 1, 2018. Accessed June 18, 2024. www.eatright.org/code-of-ethics-for-rdns-and-ndtrs

2. Deloitte Access Economics. *The Social and Economic Cost of Eating Disorders in the United States of America: A Report for the Strategic Training Initiative for the Prevention of Eating Disorders and the Academy for Eating Disorders.* June 2020. Accessed June 18, 2024. www.hsph.harvard.edu/striped/report-economic-costs-of-eating-disorders
3. Murray SB, Pila E, Griffiths S, Le Grange D. When illness severity and research dollars do not align: are we overlooking eating disorders? *World Psychiatry.* 2017;16(3):321. doi:10.1002/wps.20465
4. Coffino JA, Udo T, Grilo CM. Rates of help-seeking in US adults with lifetime DSM-5 eating disorders: prevalence across diagnoses and differences by sex and ethnicity/race. *Mayo Clin Proc.* 2019;94(8):1415-1426. doi:10.1016/j.mayocp.2019.02.030
5. Sonneville KR, Lipson SK. Disparities in eating disorder diagnosis and treatment according to weight status, race/ethnicity, socioeconomic background, and sex among college students. *Int J Eat Disord.* 2018;51(6):518-526. doi:10.1002/eat.22846
6. Marques L, Alegria M, Becker AE, et al. Comparative prevalence, correlates of impairment, and service utilization for eating disorders across US ethnic groups: implications for reducing ethnic disparities in health care access for eating disorders. *Int J Eat Disord.* 2011;44(5):412-420. doi:10.1002/eat.20787
7. Bartlett BA, Mitchell KS. Eating disorders in military and veteran men and women: a systematic review. *Int J Eat Disord.* 2015;48(8):1057-1069. doi:10.1002/eat.22454
8. Striegel-Moore RH, Rosselli F, Holtzman N, Dierker L, Becker AE, Swaney G. Behavioral symptoms of eating disorders in Native Americans: results from the ADD Health Survey Wave III. *Int J Eat Disord.* 2011;44(6):561-566. doi:10.1002/eat.20894
9. Diemer EW, Grant JD, Munn-Chernoff MA, Patterson DA, Duncan AE. Gender identity, sexual orientation, and eating-related pathology in a national sample of college students. *J Adolesc Health.* 2015;57(2):144-149. doi:10.1016/j.jadohealth.2015.03.003
10. Huryk KM, Drury CR, Loeb KL. Diseases of affluence? A systematic review of the literature on socioeconomic diversity in eating disorders. *Eat Behav.* 2021;43:101548. doi:10.1016/j.eatbeh.2021.101548
11. Halbeisen G, Brandt G, Paslakis G. A plea for diversity in eating disorders research. *Front Psychiatry.* 2022;13:820043. doi:10.3389/fpsyt.2022.820043

12. Burke NL, Hazzard VM, Schaefer LM, Simone M, O'Flynn JL, Rodgers RF. Socioeconomic status and eating disorder prevalence: at the intersections of gender identity, sexual orientation, and race/ethnicity. *Psychol Med.* 2023;53(9):4255-4265. doi:10.1017/S0033291722001015
13. Cheng ZH, Perko VL, Fuller-Marashi L, Gau JM, Stice E. Ethnic differences in eating disorder prevalence, risk factors, and predictive effects of risk factors among young women. *Eat Behav.* 2019;32:23-30. doi:10.1016/j.eatbeh.2018.11.004
14. Goode RW, Cowell MM, Mazzeo SE, et al. Binge eating and binge-eating disorder in Black women: a systematic review. *Int J Eat Disord.* 2020;53(4):491-507. doi:10.1002/eat.23217
15. Stein KF, Corte C, Ronis DL. Personal identities and disordered eating behaviors in Mexican American women. *Eat Behav.* 2010;11(3):197-200. doi:10.1016/j.eatbeh.2010.02.001
16. Smart R, Tsong Y. Weight, body dissatisfaction, and disordered eating: Asian American women's perspectives. *Asian Am J Psychology.* 2014;5(4). doi:10.1037/a0035599
17. Kinzl JF, Traweger CM, Trefalt E, Mangweth B, Biebl W. Dietitians: are they a risk group for eating disorders? *Eur Eat Disord Rev.* 1999:7:62-67.
18. Worobey J, Schoenfeld D. Eating disordered behavior in dietetics students and students in other majors. *J Am Diet Assoc.* 1999;99(9):1100-1102. doi:10.1016/S0002-8223(99)00264-3
19. Hughes R, Desbrow B. Aspiring dietitians study: a pre-enrollment study of students' motivations, awareness, and expectations relating to careers in nutrition and dietetics. *Nutr Diet.* 2005;62:106-109. doi:10.1111/j.1747-0080.2005.00015.x
20. Setnick J. Interventions used in nutrition counseling for eating disorder treatment: survey results. *SCAN's Pulse.* 2012;31(3).
21. Setnick J, Meseck K, Tackett J, Quatromoni P. A survey of registered dietitian nutritionists who provide care to clients with eating disorders: implications for education, training and clinical practic. *J Crit Diet.* 2022;6(2):1923-1237.
22. Trammell EL, Reed D, Boylan M. Education and practice gaps of registered dietitian nutritionists working with clients with eating disorders. *Top Clin Nutr.* 2016;31(1):73-85.
23. Heafala A, Ball L, Rundle-Thiele S, Mitchell LJ. "Through education, we can make change": a design thinking approach to entry-level dietetics education regarding eating disorders. *Nutr Diet.* doi:10.1111/1747-0080.12885

24. Hackert AN, Kniskern MA, Beasley TM. Academy of Nutrition and Dietetics: Revised 2020 Standards of Practice and Standards of Professional Performance for Registered Dietitian Nutritionists (Competent, Proficient, and Expert) in Eating Disorders. *J Acad Nutr Diet.* 2020;120(11):1902-1919.e54. doi:10.1016/j.jand.2020.07.014

25. International Association of Eating Disorder Professionals. *The CEDRD in Eating Disorder Care.* 2015.

26. Mahr F, Farahmand P, Bixler EO, et al. A national survey of eating disorder training. *Int J Eat Disord.* 2015;48(4):443-445. doi:10.1002/eat.22335

27. Sloan R. The role of the registered dietitian in eating disorder treatment: a reality check. *SCAN's Pulse.* 2011;30(4):11-12.

28. Reiter CS, Graves L. Nutrition therapy for eating disorders. *Nutr Clin Pract.* 2010;25(2):122-136. doi:10.1177/0884533610361606

CHAPTER 2

Eating Disorder Types and Origins

Medical and mental health providers as well as insurance organizations use the American Psychiatric Association (APA) *Diagnostic and Statistical Manual of Mental Disorders, 5th Edition, Text Revision* (*DSM-5-TR*) and World Health Organization (WHO) *International Classification of Diseases, Tenth Revision, Clinical Modification* (*ICD-10-CM*) systems for classifying eating disorders.

The *DSM-5-TR* and *ICD-10-CM* include six individually coded eating disorder diagnoses, five eating disorders grouped under an other specified feeding and eating disorders diagnostic code, and an unspecified feeding and eating disorder code.[1] Each of these has its own diagnostic and remission criteria, subtypes if applicable, and severity specifiers.*

The eating disorders with individual codes are:

- anorexia nervosa (AN),
- bulimia nervosa (BN),
- binge-eating disorder (BED),
- rumination disorder (RD),
- pica (P),
- avoidant/restrictive food intake disorder (ARFID).

---

* In 2024, the Centers for Disease Control and Prevention required *DSM-5-TR* diagnoses to exactly match *ICD-10-CM* diagnoses. This was accomplished by changing eating disorder severity ratings from optional to required and giving each level of severity its own new code.

The eating disorders included in the umbrella category other specified feeding and eating disorders (OSFED) are:

- purging disorder (PD),
- night eating syndrome (NES),
- "atypical" anorexia,
- bulimia "of low frequency or limited duration," and
- binge-eating disorder "of low frequency or limited duration."

OSFED represents multiple conditions, making it ill-suited for a discussion of specific nutrition care planning. For the remainder of this book, all OSFED conditions will be referenced by their individual names, AN, BN, BED, PD, or NES.

Expert Insight

The eating disorders in the OSFED category should not be considered less severe than the others but are less acknowledged. They carry the same risks and warrant the same urgency for treatment.[2]

Another umbrella diagnosis is unspecified feeding and eating disorders: a name and code for "other" situations. It may be used by a provider who is unable to determine a patient's specific eating issue, or when the eating disorder takes the form of chewing and spitting of food or an unhealthy fixation on "correct" or "pure" eating, called orthorexia (ON).[3]

Boxes 2.1 to 2.7 provide the *DSM-5-TR* diagnostic criteria.

BOX 2.1 Anorexia Nervosa Diagnostic Criteria

A. Restriction of energy intake relative to requirements, leading to a significantly low body weight in the context of age, sex, developmental trajectory, and physical health. *Significantly low weight* is defined as a weight that is less than minimally normal or, for children and adolescents, less than that minimally expected.

B. Intense fear of gaining weight or of becoming fat, or persistent behavior that interferes with weight gain, even though at a significantly low weight.

C. Disturbance in the way in which one's body weight or shape is experienced, undue influence of body weight or shape on self-evaluation, or persistent lack of recognition of the seriousness of the current low body weight.

Specify whether:

Restricting type: During the last 3 months, the individual has not engaged in recurrent episodes of binge-eating or purging behavior (i.e., self-induced vomiting or the misuse of laxatives, diuretics, or enemas). This subtype describes presentations in which weight loss is accomplished primarily through dieting, fasting, and/or excessive exercise.

Binge-eating/purging type: During the last 3 months, the individual has engaged in recurrent episodes of binge-eating or purging behavior (i.e., self-induced vomiting or the misuse of laxatives, diuretics, or enemas).

Specify if:

In partial remission: After full criteria for anorexia nervosa were previously met, Criterion A (low body weight) has not been met for a sustained period, but either Criterion B (intense fear of gaining weight or becoming fat or behavior that interferes with weight gain) or Criterion C (disturbances in self-perception of weight and shape) is still met.

In full remission: After full criteria for anorexia nervosa were previously met, none of the criteria have been met for a sustained period of time.

Specify current severity:

The minimum level of severity is based, for adults, on current body mass index (BMI) (see below) or, for children and adolescents, on BMI percentile. The ranges below are derived from World Health Organization categories for thinness in adults; for children and adolescents, corresponding BMI percentiles should be used. The level of severity may be increased to reflect clinical symptoms, the degree of functional disability, and the need for supervision.

BOX 2.1 Anorexia Nervosa Diagnostic Criteria (cont.)

Mild: BMI $\geq$ 17 kg/m^2

Moderate: BMI 16-16.99 kg/m^2

Severe: BMI 15-15.99 kg/m^2

Extreme: BMI < 15 kg/m^2

Coding note: The *ICD-10-CM* code depends on the subtype and the current severity/remission status (see below).

Restricting type	Binge-eating/purging type
F50.010 Mild	F50.020 Mild
F50.011 Moderate	F50.021 Moderate
F50.012 Severe	F50.022 Severe
F50.013 Extreme	F50.023 Extreme
F50.014 In partial remission	F50.024 In partial remission
F50.014 In full remission	F50.024 In full remission
F50.019 Unspecified	F50.029 Unspecified

BOX 2.2 Bulimia Nervosa Diagnostic Criteria

A. Recurrent episodes of binge eating. An episode of binge eating is characterized by both of the following:
   1. Eating, in a discrete period of time (e.g., within any 2-hour period), an amount of food that is definitely larger than what most individuals would eat in a similar period of time under similar circumstances.
   2. A sense of lack of control over eating during the episode (e.g., a feeling that one cannot stop eating or control what or how much one is eating).

B. Recurrent inappropriate compensatory behaviors in order to prevent weight gain, such as self-induced vomiting; misuse of laxatives, diuretics, or other medications; fasting; or excessive exercise.

Continued on next page

BOX 2.2 Bulimia Nervosa Diagnostic Criteria (cont.)

C. The binge eating and inappropriate compensatory behaviors both occur, on average, at least once a week for 3 months.
D. Self-evaluation is unduly influenced by body shape and weight.
E. The disturbance does not occur exclusively during episodes of anorexia nervosa.

Coding note: The *ICD-10-CM* code depends on the current severity/remission status specifier (see below). Code **F50.20** when current severity/remission status of bulimia nervosa is not specified.

Specify if:

F50.25 In partial remission: After full criteria for bulimia nervosa were previously met, some, but not all, of the criteria have been met for a sustained period of time.

F50.25 In full remission: After full criteria for bulimia nervosa were previously met, none of the criteria have been met for a sustained period of time.

Specify current severity:

The minimum level of severity is based on the frequency of inappropriate compensatory behaviors (see below). The level of severity may be increased to reflect other symptoms and the degree of functional disability.

F50.21 Mild: An average of 1-3 episodes of inappropriate compensatory behaviors per week.

F50.22 Moderate: An average of 4-7 episodes of inappropriate compensatory behaviors per week.

F50.23 Severe: An average of 8-13 episodes of inappropriate compensatory behaviors per week.

F50.24 Extreme: An average of 14 or more episodes of inappropriate compensatory behaviors per week.

F50.20 Unspecified

BOX 2.3 Binge-Eating Disorder Diagnostic Criteria

A. Recurrent episodes of binge eating. An episode of binge eating is characterized by both of the following:
   1. Eating, in a discrete period of time (e.g., within any 2-hour period), an amount of food that is definitely larger than what most people would eat in a similar period of time under similar circumstances.
   2. A sense of lack of control over eating during the episode (e.g., a feeling that one cannot stop eating or control what or how much one is eating).
B. The binge-eating episodes are associated with three (or more) of the following:
   1. Eating much more rapidly than normal.
   2. Eating until feeling uncomfortably full.
   3. Eating large amounts of food when not feeling physically hungry.
   4. Eating alone because of feeling embarrassed by how much one is eating.
   5. Feeling disgusted with oneself, depressed, or very guilty afterward.
C. Marked distress regarding binge eating is present.
D. The binge eating occurs, on average, at least once a week for 3 months.
E. The binge eating is not associated with the recurrent use of inappropriate compensatory behavior as in bulimia nervosa and does not occur exclusively during the course of bulimia nervosa or anorexia nervosa.

Coding note: The *ICD-10-CM* code depends on the current severity/remission status specifier (see below). Code **F50.819** if the current severity/remission status of binge-eating disorder is not specified.

Specify if:

F50.814 In partial remission: After full criteria for binge-eating disorder were previously met, binge eating occurs at an average frequency of less than one episode per week for a sustained period of time.

F50.814 In full remission: After full criteria for binge-eating disorder were previously met, none of the criteria have been met for a sustained period of time.

Specify current severity:

The minimum level of severity is based on the frequency of episodes of binge eating (see below). The level of severity may be increased to reflect other symptoms and the degree of functional disability.

Continued on next page

BOX 2.3 Binge-Eating Disorder Diagnostic Criteria (cont.)

F50.810 Mild: 1-3 binge-eating episodes per week.

F50.811 Moderate: 4-7 binge-eating episodes per week.

F50.812 Severe: 8-13 binge-eating episodes per week.

F50.813 Extreme: 14 or more binge-eating episodes per week.

F50.819 Unspecified

BOX 2.4 Rumination Disorder Diagnostic Criteria

A. Repeated regurgitation of food over a period of at least 1 month. Regurgitated food may be re-chewed, re-swallowed, or spit out.
B. The repeated regurgitation is not attributable to an associated gastrointestinal or other medical condition (e.g., gastroesophageal reflux, pyloric stenosis).
C. The eating disturbance does not occur exclusively during the course of anorexia nervosa, bulimia nervosa, binge-eating disorder, or avoidant/restrictive food intake disorder.
D. If the symptoms occur in the context of another mental disorder (e.g., intellectual developmental disorder [intellectual disability] or another neurodevelopmental disorder), they are sufficiently severe to warrant additional clinical attention.

Coding note: The *ICD-10-CM* codes for rumination disorder are **F98.21** in infants, children, and adolescents and **F50.84** in adults.

Specify if:

In remission: After full criteria for rumination disorder were previously met, the criteria have not been met for a sustained period of time.

BOX 2.5 Pica Diagnostic Criteria

A. Persistent eating of nonnutritive, nonfood substances over a period of at least 1 month.
B. The eating of nonnutritive, nonfood substances is inappropriate to the developmental level of the individual.
C. The eating behavior is not part of a culturally supported or socially normative practice.
D. If the eating behavior occurs in the context of another mental disorder (e.g., intellectual developmental disorder [intellectual disability], autism spectrum disorder, schizophrenia) or medical condition (including pregnancy), it is sufficiently severe to warrant additional clinical attention.

Coding note: The *ICD-10-CM* codes for pica are **F98.3** in children and adolescents and **F50.83** in adults.

Specify if:

In remission: After full criteria for pica were previously met, the criteria have not been met for a sustained period of time.

BOX 2.6 Avoidant/Restrictive Food Intake Disorder (ARFID) Diagnostic Criteria

A. An eating or feeding disturbance (e.g., apparent lack of interest in eating or food; avoidance based on the sensory characteristics of food; concern about aversive consequences of eating) associated with one (or more) of the following:
   1. Significant weight loss (or failure to achieve expected weight gain or faltering growth in children).
   2. Significant nutritional deficiency.
   3. Dependence on enteral feeding or oral nutritional supplements.
   4. Marked interference with psychosocial functioning.
B. The disturbance is not better explained by lack of available food or by an associated culturally sanctioned practice.

Continued on next page

BOX 2.6 Avoidant/Restrictive Food Intake Disorder (ARFID) Diagnostic Criteria (cont.)

C. The eating disturbance does not occur exclusively during the course of anorexia nervosa or bulimia nervosa, and there is no evidence of a disturbance in the way in which one's body weight or shape is experienced.

D. The eating disturbance is not attributable to a concurrent medical condition or not better explained by another mental disorder. When the eating disturbance occurs in the context of another condition or disorder, the severity of the eating disturbance exceeds that routinely associated with the condition or disorder and warrants additional clinical attention.

Specify if:

In remission: After full criteria for avoidant/restrictive food intake disorder were previously met, the criteria have not been met for a sustained period of time.

BOX 2.7 Other Specified Feeding or Eating Disorder (OSFED) Diagnostic Criteria

This category applies to presentations in which symptoms characteristic of a feeding and eating disorder that cause clinically significant distress or impairment in social, occupational, or other important areas of functioning predominate but do not meet the full criteria for any of the disorders in the feeding and eating disorders diagnostic class. The other specified feeding or eating disorder category is used in situations in which the clinician chooses to communicate the specific reason that the presentation does not meet the criteria for any specific feeding and eating disorder. This is done by recording "other specified feeding or eating disorder" followed by the specific reason (e.g., "bulimia nervosa of low frequency"). Examples of presentations that can be specified using the "other specified" designation include the following:

1. Atypical anorexia nervosa: All the criteria for anorexia nervosa are met, except that despite significant weight loss, the individual's weight is within or above the normal range. Individuals with atypical anorexia nervosa may experience many of the physiological complications associated with anorexia nervosa (Moskowitz and Weiselberg 2017; Peebles et al. 2010; Sawyer et al. 2016).

BOX 2.7 Other Specified Feeding or Eating Disorder (OSFED) Diagnostic Criteria (cont.)

2. Bulimia nervosa (of low frequency and/or limited duration): All of the criteria for bulimia nervosa are met, except that the binge eating and inappropriate compensatory behaviors occur, on average, less than once a week and/or for less than 3 months.
3. Binge-eating disorder (of low frequency and/or limited duration): All of the criteria for binge-eating disorder are met, except that the binge eating occurs, on average, less than once a week and/or for less than 3 months.
4. Purging disorder: Recurrent purging behavior to influence weight or shape (e.g., self-induced vomiting; misuse of laxatives, diuretics, or other medications) in the absence of binge eating.
5. Night eating syndrome: Recurrent episodes of night eating, as manifested by eating after awakening from sleep or by excessive food consumption after the evening meal. There is awareness and recall of the eating. The night eating is not better explained by external influences such as changes in the individual's sleep-wake cycle or by local social norms. The night eating causes significant distress and/or impairment in functioning. The disordered pattern of eating is not better explained by binge-eating disorder or another mental disorder, including substance use, and is not attributable to another medical condition or to an effect of medication.

Origins of Dysfunctional Eating Behavior

Dysfunctional eating behaviors are, by definition, harmful, so why do they start and why do they persist? Researchers have many theories but no clear answers. Genetic studies hold promise, but no answers yet. Generalizations are flawed as there are exceptions to everything. It is likely that multiple factors play a role, and their contributions vary for each person. It is difficult to even define when eating disorders start. "Age of onset" usually means age at diagnosis, but problems could have been occurring for years prior.

What this means in practice is that each patient is an *n* of one. The practitioner should not hold any assumptions based on past patients and there should be no reliance on standard protocol. The origin of each eating disorder is unique, and it may be impossible to find. Identify and solve the contributing factors and the eating disorder may improve ... or it may not. Can't find any contributing factors? Treat the symptoms anyway. Although there are as many paths to eating disorders as there are individuals experiencing them, contributing factors tend to fit into the four groups summarized in Box 2.8.

BOX 2.8 Origins of Dysfunctional Eating Behavior (DEB) Model

Biology-based DEB

Caused by	Genes Epigenetics Conditions that cause brain damage Conditions that cause or require alterations in metabolism, diet, or weight
Looks like or can co-occur with	Obsessive-compulsive disorder (OCD), anxiety, attention-deficit with hyperactivity disorder (ADHD), neurodivergence, pediatric acute-onset neuropsychiatric syndrome (PANS), polycystic ovary syndrome (PCOS), hypothyroid, sleep disorders, diabetes, celiac disease, food allergies, Prader-Willi syndrome, infectious disease, autoimmune disease, concussion, gastrointestinal conditions, cancer, lupus, Lyme disease, COVID-19, etc.
Treatment	Treatment is specific to underlying or co-occurring conditions Medication Brain-based interventions Nutritional rehabilitation

BOX 2.8 Origins of Dysfunctional Eating Behavior (DEB) Model (cont.)

Addiction-based DEB

Caused by	Alterations in brain chemistry due to substance use Genetic predisposition to addiction Attempts to control weight-related effects of addiction or sobriety
Looks like or can co-occur with	Substance abuse or heavy use, self-harm, process addictions, family history of alcohol abuse or addiction, chronic pain
Treatment	Specific to addiction Pharmacology Twelve-step programs such as Alcoholics Anonymous (AA), Anorexia and Bulimia Anonymous (ABA), Adult Children of Alcoholics (ACOA), Narcotics Anonymous (NA), and so on Peer support/sponsorship Support groups Nutrition education and counseling Abstinence model, based primarily on abstaining from DEB, not food

Trauma/stress-based DEB

Caused by	Alterations in brain function resulting from traumatic life events, chronic stress, perfectionism, internal or external pressures for high achievement
Looks like or can co-occur with	Post-traumatic stress disorder (PTSD), trauma history, removal from home, neglect, abandonment, disruption of living situation, tragic loss, bullying, insecure attachment, food insecurity, incarceration, chronic illness, disability, systemic racism/inequality, weight stigma, immigration

Continued on next page

BOX 2.8 Origins of Dysfunctional Eating Behavior (DEB) Model (cont.)

Trauma/stress-based DEB (continued)

Treatment	Pharmacology to treat concurrent conditions Nutritional education and counseling Eye movement desensitization and reprocessing (EMDR), somatic experiencing (SE), dialectical behavior therapy (DBT), or talk therapy Support groups Grief/loss/crisis counseling, and so on, as appropriate

Social/learned DEB

Caused by	Peer pressure Body dissatisfaction Family or cultural food practices (such as withholding food as punishment) Societal standards of attractiveness Dieting Food trends such as "cleanses" External locus of weight control such as athletic weight requirements Weight loss surgery Weight loss drugs
Looks like or can co-occur with	Chronic dieting, binge eating or drinking, weight fluctuations, low self-esteem, promiscuity
Treatment	Nutrition education and counseling Mindfulness practice Intuitive eating Media literacy Self-esteem work Family counseling

Adapted with permission from reference 4; Setnick J. *Eating Disorders Boot Camp: Training Workshop for Professionals*. 2013, rev 2017. Accessed June 19, 2024. www.eatingdisordersbootcamp.com

Biological Factors

Genes

According to the Eating Disorders Genetics Initiative, 40% to 60% of eating disorder risk is genetic,[5] but research identifying specific genes is in its infancy. Although specific gene therapies are not available, the knowledge that eating disorders are biological in nature and not character flaws or poor choices can be helpful to patients and families.[6-10]

Restriction of energy, macronutrients, and micronutrients causes cascades of biochemical and psychological changes.[11] It is not clear why some malnourished individuals develop eating disorders while others do not. External reinforcement for weight loss may be a factor but not the only factor, as weight loss may continue past the point of social praise. Further genetic and epigenetic research will hopefully shed more light on the interaction between voluntary and involuntary starvation, malnutrition, and eating disorder development.

Individual genome testing has shown some promise in identifying mutations that result in metabolic and eating disruptions. Some of these mutations can be treated, with resulting improvement in eating disorder symptoms.[12] As investigation into specific genes, their mechanisms, and epigenetic responses continues to evolve, it will inform medical nutrition therapy (MNT) for eating disorders.

Neurochemistry and the Gut Microbiome

Researchers have studied the dysregulation of serotonin, dopamine, leptin, ghrelin, and melanocortin systems in relation to eating disorders. This is based on the hypothesis that certain eating behaviors are biochemically rewarding to certain individuals because of their effects on brain chemistry. Alterations in reward circuitry in the brain and even brain structure are being reviewed, as well as microbes and neurons present in the digestive system.

Because research is usually conducted after the onset of eating disorders, it does not differentiate between dysregulation that was present before (and therefore may have contributed to) the eating disorder vs dysregulation caused after the fact by dysfunctional eating behaviors or malnutrition. Although to date there are no overarching conclusions, psychopharmacology, MNT, and behavioral strategies that improve or address brain chemistry can be effective in some cases when used on a trial-and-error basis.

Psychiatric Disorders

Eating disorders often co-occur with symptoms of other psychiatric conditions, such as anxiety, depression, obsessive-compulsive disorder,[13] attention-deficit hyperactivity disorder, personality disorders, suicidality, and nonsuicidal self-injury.[14-17] In some cases, one condition presents first and appears to cause the other. In other cases, it seems that one precursor causes both conditions, which then exist side-by-side or exacerbate each other. Currently, best practice is to treat both or all conditions rather than assuming that treating one will resolve the other(s), although sometimes that does happen.

Chronic Medical Conditions

Any medical illness or diagnosis that requires a change in dietary intake can start the process toward dysfunctional eating. In some cases, the pathway seems deceptively simple: a dietary change leads to metabolic and neurochemical changes that lead to an eating disorder. In other cases, depression or anxiety about the diagnosis is an intermediary factor that then leads to an eating disorder. There may be more complex connections as well. One underlying genetic factor may contribute to both the medical condition and the eating disorder, as suggested by the frequent co-occurrence of anorexia nervosa and autoimmune diseases.[18] Strong connections have been found between anorexia nervosa and celiac disease, type 1 diabetes, and inflammatory bowel disease, but the exact mechanisms are unknown.[18-21]

Other chronic medical conditions that commonly co-occur with eating disorders include iron-deficiency anemia, polycystic ovary syndrome, menstrual dysfunction, type 2 diabetes, cancer, thyroid dysfunction, gastroparesis, and other gastrointestinal conditions.[22-25] It can be challenging to determine which came first, so as with co-occurring psychiatric conditions, best practice is to assess and treat both conditions rather than assuming that resolution of one will fix the other.

Acute Medical Conditions

Pediatric acute-onset neuropsychiatric syndrome (PANS) occurs when an illness leads to rapid development of symptoms that may include tics, developmental regression, anxiety, or food refusal that can mimic or become anorexia nervosa.[26,27] The progression of PANS is not well understood. Other acute medical conditions that can cause eating disorders are concussion (due to appetite fluctuations) and COVID-19 (due to loss of taste and smell).

Addictions

When substance or process addictions (such as compulsive gambling or gaming) co-occur with eating disorders, they can influence and reinforce each other in a bidirectional cause-and-effect loop.[28] Marijuana use can soothe nausea and also cause uncontrollable vomiting.[29] Alcohol can lower dietary inhibition, causing overeating, and can also inhibit appetite when overused. Stimulants tend to depress appetite. The neurochemical changes associated with eating disorder behaviors are similar to those induced by drugs of abuse, which may explain why someone abstaining from their addiction may find dysfunctional eating behaviors soothing. Best practice is to address both issues concurrently if possible.

"Food addiction" is itself a term that sparks strong feelings in different camps—those who believe that food items or ingredients hold addictive capabilities, and those who believe that addiction-like symptoms are caused by food restrictions but not by the actual foods. There is evidence on both sides of the debate, suggesting that no one answer applies to everyone.[30] Some people may indeed experience addiction-like responses to food ingredients when they eat them and withdrawal symptoms when they do not, while others are able to eat all foods without negative consequences once they have dissociated the particular foods with shame and wrongdoing.[31]

Stress and Trauma

Extensive research has linked eating dysfunction to traumatic incidents, post-traumatic stress disorder, and chronic stress.[12,32-37] Traumatic events that lead to eating disorders may be related to food, as in food insecurity, receiving terrible news at a meal, or a foodborne illness; related to bodily autonomy, such as bullying, being weight-shamed by a medical provider, domestic violence, physical or sexual assault; or unrelated to either, such as a natural disaster or personal or community tragedy. Trauma-related food behaviors may develop immediately or long after the event.

Chronic or ongoing stress (ie, not linked to one specific traumatic moment in time) is another major contributor to dysfunctional eating and, as with trauma, may or may not be food related. For example, the experience of foster care can be an eating disorder trigger on its own even if food insecurity is not involved. The experience of immigration, acculturation, and other aspects of being in a new place, such as learning a new language, are very stressful. Parts of the immigration and acculturation journey may cause specific food difficulties. The stress of any of these experiences can trigger dysfunctional eating behaviors as an attempt at self-medication that soothes disrupted brain chemistry.

Additional examples of ongoing stress that are not food-related yet may cause eating dysfunction include lack of access to gender-affirming care or refusal of medical procedures due to weight requirements. When any individual is denied medical care, they may experience depression and distress that can disrupt nutrition. When the denial of medical care means that an individual must continue to live in chronic pain or gender dysphoria, the effects can be intensified.

In addition, the impact of social determinants of health on stress levels and thus eating disorder development cannot be overstated. Food insecurity, systemic racism, ableism, unsafe living conditions, military service, immigrant status, homelessness, incarceration, health care disparities, weight surveillance, and stigma—all of these disproportionately affect the very same communities and groups that have been historically and systematically excluded from eating disorder research and treatment. And even when included, the chronic stress of being in a marginalized group can impair eating disorder treatment by impacting interoceptive awareness and gastrointestinal function.

It is likely that there are multiple metabolic pathways from acute or chronic stress to eating disorder, but exact mechanisms are as yet unknown. Dysfunctional eating and compensatory behaviors (eg, self-induced vomiting, laxative abuse, excessive exercise, and nonsuicidal self-injury) cause neurochemical changes that can soothe distress, serve as a distraction, provide a temporary feeling of well-being, or prompt a dissociative state. Behaviors that appear from an outside perspective to be harmful can serve as a method of self-soothing or self-medication to the individual practicing them. Appropriate treatment for a stress-induced eating disorder addresses eating behaviors while providing skills to remove or cope with the underlying stressor(s).

Social and Cultural Pressures

Weight bias (the belief that body size determines health), weight stigma (treating larger people differently), and diet culture (the belief that we need external direction to eat correctly) are significant contributors to dysfunctional eating. Individuals are constantly encouraged to eat less and weigh less as dictated by fashion, social media, advertising, health care, school, sports, employers, and more.

Outside of the eating disorder field, following restrictive diets, taking daily weights, and wearing fitness trackers signal "being health-conscious" or "taking care of yourself" rather than evidence of body surveillance and the oppression of physical appearance. Comments about bodies and weight changes are considered normal and are expected. Individuals who are fat, superfat, or infinifat experience fatphobia in the forms of discrimination, hostility, bullying, and exclusion. Medical research ignores healthy fat people and focuses on body shrinkage, ignoring that for most individuals weight-loss methods are unsustainable and may actually damage health. In sadly familiar cases, medical care is withheld in favor of weight loss, leading to deterioration and in some cases, death.

Social and cultural pressures are such significant factors in the creation and perpetuation of dysfunctional eating behaviors that every registered dietitian nutritionist (RDN) should strive to cleanse their work environment of body-shaming messages and usage of weight as a proxy for health. We should emphasize that people of all shapes, sizes, and descriptions are worthy and deserving of care; recognize that weight stigma is connected to other forms of systemic oppression such as racism and ableism; and investigate our own biases against fatness to ensure that we are not adding to the problem.

Universal Precautions

Because the possible factors that cause and contribute to eating disorders are so broad in scope and yet so unknown in specificity, it is crucial that RDNs enter each patient interaction with the knowledge that—whether diagnosed, discussed, or even known to the individual—every human carries the potential for dysfunctional eating behavior. Similar to the standard precautions widely used in health care settings for infection control, the Universal Precautions for Dietitians stem from the assertion that risk is everywhere, even when not previously ascertained or identified.[4] This means that, regardless of the setting in which it takes place, regardless of a patient's diagnoses, regardless of the RDN's personal feelings about an individual, all MNT should be trauma-informed, all MNT should be weight-inclusive, and all MNT should prioritize harm reduction, beneficence, autonomy, and justice in accordance with our Code of Ethics.[38-41]

References

1. American Psychiatric Association. Feeding and eating disorders. In: *Diagnostic and Statistical Manual of Mental Disorders*. 5th rev ed. 2022:371-397.
2. Brennan C, Illingworth S, Cini E, Bhakta D. Medical instability in typical and atypical adolescent anorexia nervosa: a systematic review and meta-analysis. *J Eat Disord*. 2023;11(1):58. doi:10.1186/s40337-023-00779-y
3. Donini LM, Barrada JR, Barthels F, et al. A consensus document on definition and diagnostic criteria for orthorexia nervosa. *Eat Weight Disord*. 2022;27(8):3695-3711. doi:10.1007/s40519-022-01512-5

4. Setnick J. *Eating Disorders Boot Camp: Training Workshop for Professionals*. 2013, rev 2017. Accessed June 19, 2024. www.eatingdisordersbootcamp.com
5. Eating Disorders Genetics Initiative. 2021. Accessed June 19, 2024. http://edgi.org
6. Yilmaz Z, Hardaway JA, Bulik CM. Genetics and epigenetics of eating disorders. *Adv Genomics Genet*. 2015;5:131-150. doi:10.2147/AGG.S55776
7. Klump KL, Burt SA, McGue M, Iacono WG. Changes in genetic and environmental influences on disordered eating across adolescence: a longitudinal twin study. *Arch Gen Psychiatry*. 2007;64(12):1409-1415. doi:10.1001/archpsyc.64.12.1409
8. Wade TD, Bulik CM, Sullivan PF, Neale MC, Kendler KS. The relation between risk factors for binge eating and bulimia nervosa: a population-based female twin study. *Health Psychol*. 2000;19(2):115-123. doi:10.1037/0278-6133.19.2.115
9. Strober M, Freeman R, Lampert C, Diamond J, Kaye W. Controlled family study of anorexia nervosa and bulimia nervosa: evidence of shared liability and transmission of partial syndromes. *Am J Psychiatry*. 2000;157(3):393-401. doi:10.1176/appi.ajp.157.3.393
10. Grice DE, Halmi KA, Fichter MM, et al. Evidence for a susceptibility gene for anorexia nervosa on chromosome 1. *Am J Hum Genet*. 2002;70(3):787-792. doi:10.1086/339250
11. Kalm LM, Semba RD. They starved so that others be better fed: remembering Ancel Keys and the Minnesota experiment. *J Nutr*. 2005;135(6):1347-1352. doi:10.1093/jn/135.6.1347
12. Lutter M. *GIFTED: Genetic Information for Treating Eating Disorders*. Michael Lutter; 2023.
13. Trottier K, Wonderlich SA, Monson CM, Crosby RD, Olmsted MP. Investigating posttraumatic stress disorder as a psychological maintaining factor of eating disorders. *Int J Eat Disord*. 2016;49(5):455-457. doi:10.1002/eat.22516
14. Sansone RA, Sansone LA. Personality pathology and its influence on eating disorders. *Innov Clin Neurosci*. 2011;8(3):14-18.
15. Kiekens G, Claes L. Non-suicidal self-injury and eating disordered behaviors: an update on what we do and do not know. *Curr Psychiatry Rep*. 2020;22(12):68. doi:10.1007/s11920-020-01191-y
16. Reinblatt SP. Are eating disorders related to attention deficit/hyperactivity disorder? *Curr Treat Options Psychiatry*. 2015;2(4):402-412. doi:10.1007/s40501-015-0060-7
17. Puccio F, Fuller-Tyszkiewicz M, Ong D, Krug I. A systematic review and meta-analysis on the longitudinal relationship between eating pathology and depression. *Int J Eat Disord*. 2016;49(5):439-454. doi:10.1002/eat.22506

18. Raevuori A, Haukka J, Vaarala O, et al. The increased risk for autoimmune diseases in patients with eating disorders. *PLoS One*. 2014;9(8):e104845. doi:10.1371/journal.pone.0104845

19. Mårild K, Størdal K, Bulik CM, et al. Celiac disease and anorexia nervosa: a nationwide study. *Pediatrics*. 2017;139(5):e20164367. doi:10.1542/peds.2016-4367

20. Hanlan ME, Griffith J, Patel N, Jaser SS. Eating disorders and disordered eating in type 1 diabetes: prevalence, screening, and treatment options. *Curr Diab Rep*. doi:10.1007/s11892-013-0418-4

21. Riehl ME, Scarlata K. Understanding disordered eating risks in patients with gastrointestinal conditions. *J Acad Nutr Diet*. 2022;122(3):491-499. doi:10.1016/j.jand.2021.03.001

22. Nicolau J, Simó R, Sanchís P, et al. Eating disorders are frequent among type 2 diabetic patients and are associated with worse metabolic and psychological outcomes: results from a cross-sectional study in primary and secondary care settings. *Acta Diabetol*. 2015;52(6):1037-1044. doi:10.1007/s00592-015-0742-z

23. Hossein SA, Bahrami M, Mohamadirizi S, Paknahad Z. Investigation of eating disorders in cancer patients and its relevance with body image. *Iran J Nurs Midwifery Res*. 2015;20(3):327-333.

24. Michels N, De Backer F, Dimakopoulou M, Mane K, Indave I, Huybrechts I. Eating disorders and the risk of developing cancer: a systematic review. *Eat Weight Disord*. 2021;26(4):1021-1035. doi:10.1007/s40519-020-01020-4

25. Yahya AH, Khawaja S, Williams PS, Naguib M. Binge eating disorder and type 2 diabetes: epidemiology and treatment approaches. *Prog. Neurol. Psychiatry*. 2022;26(2):33-37. doi:10.1002/pnp.749

26. Pallanti S, Di Ponzio M. PANDAS/PANS in the COVID-19 Age: autoimmunity and Epstein-Barr virus reactivation as trigger agents? *Children (Basel)*. 2023;10(4):648. doi:10.3390/children10040648

27. Pavone P, Ceccarelli M, Marino S, et al. SARS-CoV-2 related paediatric acute-onset neuropsychiatric syndrome. *Lancet Child Adolesc Health*. 2021;5(6):e19-e21. doi:10.1016/S2352-4642(21)00135-8

28. Kalra SP, Kalra PS. Overlapping and interactive pathways regulating appetite and craving. *J Addict Dis*. 2004;23(3):5-21. doi:10.1300/J069v23n03_02

29. Venkatesan T, Levinthal DJ, Li BUK, et al. Role of chronic cannabis use: cyclic vomiting syndrome vs cannabinoid hyperemesis syndrome. *Neurogastroenterol Motil*. 2019;31:Suppl 2(Suppl 2):e13606. doi:10.1111/nmo.13606

30. Wiss D, Brewerton T. Separating the signal from the noise: how psychiatric diagnoses can help discern food addiction from dietary restraint. *Nutrients.* 2020;12(10):2937. doi:10.3390/nu12102937
31. Wiss D. Clinical considerations of ultra-processed food addiction across weight classes: an eating disorder treatment and care perspective. *Curr Addict Rep.* 2022;9(4):255-267. doi:10.1007/s40429-022-00411-0
32. Hardaway JA, Crowley NA, Bulik CM, Kash TL. Integrated circuits and molecular components for stress and feeding: implications for eating disorders. *Genes Brain Behav.* 2015;14(1):85-97. doi:10.1111/gbb.12185
33. Rantala MJ, Luoto S, Krama T, Krams I. Eating disorders: an evolutionary psychoneuroimmunological approach. *Front Psychol.* 2019;10:2200. doi:10.3389/fpsyg.2019.02200
34. Brewerton T. The links between PTSD and eating disorders. *Psychiatric Times.* 2008;25(6).May 2, 2008. Accessed June 12, 2023. www.psychiatric times.com/view/links-between-ptsd-and-eating-disorders
35. Mitchell KS, Mazzeo SE, Schlesinger MR, Brewerton TD, Smith BN. Comorbidity of partial and subthreshold PTSD among men and women with eating disorders in the national comorbidity survey-replication study. *Int J Eat Disord.* 2012;45(3):307-315. doi:10.1002/eat.20965
36. Kessler RC, Sonnega A, Bromet E, Hughes M, Nelson CB. Posttraumatic stress disorder in the National Comorbidity Survey. *Arch Gen Psychiatry.* 1995;52(12):1048-1060. doi:10.1001/archpsyc.1995.03950240066012
37. Dansky BS, Brewerton TD, Kilpatrick DG, O'Neil PM. The National Women's Study: relationship of victimization and posttraumatic stress disorder to bulimia nervosa. *Int J Eat Disord.* 1997;21(3):213-228. doi:10 .1002/(sici)1098-108x(199704)21:3<213::aid-eat2>3.0.co;2-n
38. Academy of Nutrition and Dietetics, Commission on Dietetic Registration. Code of Ethics for the Nutrition and Dietetics Profession. June 1, 2018. Accessed June 19, 2024. www.eatright.org/-/media/files /eatright/coeforthenutritionanddieteticsprofession.pdf
39. Hawk M, Coulter RWS, Egan JE, et al. Harm reduction principles for healthcare settings. *Harm Reduct J.* 2017;14(1):70. doi:10.1186/s12954-017 -0196-4
40. Dada J. Weight-inclusive care: evidence and best practices. *Today's Dietitian.* 2020. Accessed July 22, 2024. www.todaysdietitian.com/pdf /courses/DadaWeightInclusive.pdf
41. Center for Health Care Strategies. What is trauma-informed care? 2024. Accessed July 22, 2024. www.traumainformedcare.chcs.org/what-is -trauma-informed-care

CHAPTER 3

Nutrition Assessment for Eating Disorders

Inpatient vs Outpatient Settings

The most significant difference in performing a nutrition assessment in different levels of care is the amount of information available. In an outpatient setting, a registered dietitian nutritionist (RDN) often has only the patient's self-report to rely on, sometimes with input from another care provider or support partner. In an inpatient or residential setting, an RDN can usually speak with other care providers who may have observed a patient's mealtime behavior, mood, or demeanor, plus access to additional details such as psychological test results and previous medical records. (Refer to Chapter 8 for more information on the different levels of eating disorder care.)

In a specialty treatment center, behavioral health facility, or hospital, your thorough nutrition assessment of a patient with dysfunctional eating will help determine the care plan and the goals set by the treatment team and should be performed as soon as is reasonable after admission. Be aware of facility protocols and state or certification requirements governing the time frame for nutrition assessment so that you can meet expectations.

Expert Insight

Because dangerous eating behaviors are often not treated or diagnosed in their early stages, someone may seek outpatient care when they really need inpatient or emergency treatment. Keep in mind that outpatient or ambulatory status does not automatically indicate that a person is safe or medically stable.

Patients who are medically unstable may require nutrition support on an emergency basis before a more thorough nutrition assessment can be performed, and patients who are extremely malnourished, uncooperative, or hostile (such as those who are hospitalized against their will) may need time to adjust before meeting productively with you. When faced with a situation in which you cannot gather information from the patient directly, draft a preliminary nutrition assessment using information available to you from medical records, family members, support partners, and other providers.

In either setting, as you gather information for your assessment, you may find differences of opinion regarding severity, frequency, and duration of symptoms. Document your findings even if they are inconclusive, as a full nutrition assessment may require several meetings with the patient or their support partners.

Interviewing Patients

In an ideal world, your patients would welcome your assistance and answer all your questions helpfully. In reality, there are many reasons why someone may not be forthcoming with information—resenting needing help, regretting their choice to enter treatment, worrying about retaliation for sharing "family secrets," discomfort speaking with a stranger, a past bad experience with a different dietitian, or their own shame. Try not to take this personally, and if you do not gather as much information as you would have hoped, consider that your first meeting was at least a step toward building a trusting bond. If your initial meeting with a patient is the first time they have ever spoken about their eating with a professional—or with anyone—respect the effort it may be taking for this person to come forward. Your nonjudgmental acceptance of however much the patient is willing to share has the potential to encourage them to continue to pursue recovery in general, and expressions of compassion and hope may be as important as the nutrition information you convey, even if they do not pursue care with you or at this time.

Expert Insight

If a patient asks you to keep their risky eating behaviors secret or refuses recommended medical care, seek advice from a supervisor or trusted colleague on how to proceed.

Appropriate Terminology and Questions

Box 3.1 lists sample questions specific to gathering information about dysfunctional eating behaviors that can be added to those you typically ask during a nutrition assessment. As with any nutrition assessment, tailor your questions to each patient's needs; it is unlikely you will ask all these questions to any one patient. Pick and choose what seems appropriate based on your preliminary knowledge of the patient's situation and adapt as you go.

Use general terminology rather than technical or eating-disorder specific language. If the patient uses terms like "binge" and "purge," ask them to elaborate or provide an example. This will limit misunderstandings and help you avoid introducing new ideas.

BOX 3.1 Sample Questions for Eating Disorder Assessment

"Can you bring me up to date on what brought you here?" If the patient denies having dysfunctional eating or states, "I'm only here because [someone else] thinks I have a problem," ask, "What is your understanding of why [that person] wanted you to be here?"

"How do you decide what, when, and how much to eat?"

"Describe your eating on a typical day." Include timing and content of meals and snacks. If the patient specifies "on a good day..." or "on a bad day ..." follow up on what, in the patient's opinion, makes eating "good" or "bad" and how often each type of day occurs. Include timing and quantities of noncaloric and nonnutritional food and beverage items, including abnormal intake of condiments, water, artificial sweeteners, coffee, chewing gum, alcohol, energy drinks, and so on.

"Are you allergic to any foods? ... Are there other foods that you don't or won't eat? ... What are the reasons you don't eat those foods?"

"Do you ever worry that you'll get out of control around food and eat much more than you intended to? ... Is it just a worry, or does it sometimes happen?"

"Can you give me an example of what you might eat that feels like way too much? ... How often does this happen?"

"What foods are your weakness? ... Do you try to avoid them? ... What happens when you are around them eventually?"

"Do you ever eat in secret? ... How is it different than eating with others?"

"Do you wake up in the middle of the night to eat? ... Do you ever wake up to find evidence of eating that surprises you?"

"Do you ever have trouble keeping your food down?"

"Do you ever enjoy eating but then feel guilty afterward? ... What happens next? ... Do you ever feel like you have to make up for what you ate?"

"Do you ever avoid eating when you're hungry?"

"Is there anything special you do with food preparation or when eating? ... Anything you can't or won't eat? Routines that you follow when preparing or plating your food or during a meal?" Examples include cutting food into many tiny pieces, reheating food during a meal, drawing out a meal for a certain length of time, eating only with certain dishware or flatware, measuring or weighing portions before eating, or eating only a certain number of items at a time (eg, everything in threes). Ask about the reason for or motivation behind these

Continued on next page

BOX 3.1 Sample Questions for Eating Disorder Assessment (cont.)

behaviors to determine if they are causing or solving problems. Individuals who are neurodivergent or disabled and those with sensory processing or neuromotor differences may use behaviors traditionally labeled as "disordered" (such as cutting food into small pieces or drinking after each bite) in a supportive or assistive way.

Ask about other dysfunctional eating behaviors not already described, such as sham eating (chewing and spitting, or otherwise pretending to eat), laxative use, compulsive weighing, and so on. Include frequency of behavior and any identifiable triggers ("Does it happen every time you eat, or only in certain situations? ... What situations cause that?").

Ask about physical activity. If applicable, include frequency, duration, and type of exercise; compulsion to exercise ("Can you miss a day of exercise?"); secrecy of exercise ("Do you ever exercise even though you're not supposed to?"); relationship between exercise and eating ("Is your eating the same on a day you exercise and a day you don't exercise?"); exercise rituals ("Is there anything specific that you do every time you exercise?"); as well as any recommendations from other health providers recommending or restricting physical activities ("Has a doctor or other provider told you to rest or stop exercising?").

Expert Insight

If you notice that a patient responds differently to questions when their support partners are present, consider asking the patient privately if they are aware of the difference. If the patient is uncomfortable speaking freely when others are present, ask the patient to share that with their mental health provider for guidance.

Some answers will require follow-up questions. When you do not know what to say, "Tell me more about that" is the perfect response. Your goal is not to gather every possible data point on a patient in the first session, but rather to obtain baseline information to inform your recommendations. Ideally you will have more opportunities to meet with this individual and continue to gather (and provide) more information each time.

Nutrition Assessment: Food-/ Nutrition-Related History

Your interview will likely touch on all categories in the Nutrition Assessment section of the Nutrition Care Process[1] (refer to Appendix A for more detail on the Nutrition Care Process). The following sections use Nutrition Care Process terminology[2] to explain how dysfunctional eating may affect the different Nutrition Assessment categories and specify appropriate referrals for non-nutrition-related findings. Note that any of these features can occur in any eating diagnosis or in the absence of a diagnosis; the diagnoses in parentheses are simply suggestions to guide further assessment in any patient exhibiting the given behavior. The following abbreviations will be utilized here:

- AN = anorexia nervosa/atypical anorexia nervosa
- ARFID = avoidant/restrictive food intake disorder
- BED = binge-eating disorder/binge-eating disorder of low frequency or limited duration
- BN = bulimia nervosa/bulimia nervosa of low frequency or limited duration
- ED = eating disorder
- NES = night eating syndrome
- ON = orthorexia nervosa
- P = pica
- PD = purging disorder
- RD = rumination disorder

Assessment of Excess Intake

Alcohol (includes binge drinking): Alcohol use can cause dysfunctional eating and nutrition deficiencies even in the absence of alcohol dependence or abuse. Examples include "drunkorexia," slang for skipping meals prior to drinking (AN, BN, BED), and "boot and rallying," meaning inducing vomiting in order to drink more (BN, PD).

Caffeine: Drinking coffee (or ingesting instant coffee crystals or coffee beans), tea, caffeinated carbonated beverages, and caffeinated "energy drinks" can result in an excessive intake of caffeine and other stimulants (Appendix C). Caffeine can depress or mask appetite (AN, BN, BED, PD), maintain energy levels in the face of insufficient caloric intake (AN, BN, PD, ARFID), compensate for poor sleep quality (NES), or propel excessive exercise (AN, BN, BED). Some patients use caffeine and other stimulants on purpose, while others are not aware that their use is affecting their appetite or increasing their anxiety.

Expert Insight

A patient who reports headaches when not using caffeine (caffeine dependence) may require a weaning protocol to prevent physical withdrawal symptoms. A patient overusing or abusing caffeine/stimulants may benefit from a medical evaluation for chronic fatigue or a psychiatric evaluation for attention-deficit with hyperactivity disorder (ADHD).

Fortified foods and supplements containing vitamins and minerals: Preoccupation with nutrient content (ON), portion control (AN, BED, BN), desire for standardization (ARFID), or lack of variety (AN, ON, ARFID) can lead to overuse of fortified foods vs produce or homemade foods. Separately, self-prescription of micronutrient supplements can lead to excess intake (AN, ON).

Substances that interfere with digestion or absorption (including fiber, fluids, and foods without available vitamins): Reliance on "filler" foods (bulky items high in insoluble fiber, such as rice cakes and bran cereal) to provide a physical feeling of fullness with few calories (AN) can cause constipation, insufficient micronutrient intake, and limited absorption of nutrients bound by fiber.

Convenience foods, preprepared meals, and foods prepared away from home (including sodium, energy-dense or high-fat foods and beverages): There are many factors to assess when a patient is reliant on convenience foods; it is not appropriate to assume that convenience food use is a problem that should be changed. Predictability, standard portion sizes, and consistency in taste and texture can be helpful for people with sensory sensitivities (ARFID). Assess for food insecurity, access to grocery stores, time constraints, safe food storage in the home (pest control, refrigeration, food safety practices), knowledge of food preparation, availability of kitchen tools and appliances, and other environmental factors before determining a course of action. Some convenience foods are specifically eaten during a binge episode, either because they are inexpensive, highly palatable, considered easy to purge, or because of guilt associated with eating them (BED, PD, BN).

Volume of food in a defined period: Assess what the patient defines as "an excessive amount of food" as well as if they experience a loss of control or shame during or after an episode (BED, BN). Are the episodes related to food insecurity or other fluctuations in food availability?

Other Factors Associated With Excess Intake

Binge-eating patterns: If a patient reports "binge eating," ask for their definition; in some cases, a "binge" may simply be more than a person intended to eat. Learn the circumstances of binge episodes—are there patterns to what, when, how much, why? Ask about what and when they last ate before a binge episode. Was it caused by an extended period without eating or not eating enough? Do the episodes interrupt the patient's sleep (NES)? Do they lead to compensatory behaviors (BN)?

> ***Expert Insight***
>
> *Binge episodes can occur within any eating disorder diagnosis, including anorexia nervosa.*

Change in way clothes fit: Compulsively or punitively trying on a certain item of clothing ("body-checking") to detect a change or lack of change in the fit can prompt dysfunctional eating behaviors. Body size change may result in discomfort for patients unable to afford new clothing.

Highly variable calorie intake: A drastically varying eating pattern ("good days" and "bad days") can lead to shame (AN, BED) and compensatory behaviors (BN, PD), and can result from food insecurity.

Assessment of Insufficient Intake

Carbohydrates and fiber: Many trendy weight-loss diets villainize "carbs," and that bad reputation has overflowed into a general fear or avoidance of them (AN, ON) and guilt after eating them (BN, BED). Alternately, many convenience foods are low in fiber, so although a patient is not purposely avoiding carbohydrates, their total intake may be low in soluble fiber, leading to constipation (ARFID).

Energy: Insufficient energy intake is a feature of every eating disorder. A 24-hour recall is not adequate to assess energy intake; ask about different days (eg, "a good day and a bad day" or "a day when you eat and a day when you don't eat").

Fluid: Assess the reason for fluid restriction. Is it related to a medical diagnosis or medication? Contaminated local water supply? An attempt to decrease body weight, prevent feeling "bloated," "full," or the need to urinate (all ED)?

Fat and essential fatty acids: Trendy diets and even legitimate dietary guidance have villainized dietary fats. Restricting dietary fat intake

Expert Insight

The RDN often must educate other disciplines that a large body size is not proof that a patient is eating adequately.

Expert Insight

Rather than recommending weight loss or dietary fat restriction to address elevated liver enzymes, consider whether fat intake is currently insufficient. If so, increased fat intake is needed.

can be a misguided attempt to lose weight or seek health, but instead it causes poor absorption of fat-soluble micronutrients, impairs essential fatty acid intake, and may affect liver function (all ED).

Food (including supplements, nutrients, vitamins, and minerals): Assessing for food preferences and variety will point to corresponding nutritional deficiencies (all ED).

Food(s) from specific food groups related to gastrointestinal (GI) symptoms: The overlap between GI disorders and eating disorders could fill its own book. Assess for any known GI conditions that can impair eating or digestion—reflux, ulcers, celiac disease, inflammatory bowel disease (ulcerative colitis, Crohn's disease), cancer, pancreatitis, gallbladder disease, etc. Assess for GI symptoms—constipation, diarrhea, excessive flatulence or burping, bloating, delayed gastric emptying, nausea, vomiting, etc. Ask if a patient's dietary restrictions are related to their GI distress (AN, ON, ARFID). Assess the timeline of GI symptoms and eating behaviors to determine if the GI distress may have been present first, in which case a GI consult is in order. If the GI symptoms seem to be resulting from the eating behaviors, they may resolve with improved nutrition, but it is not appropriate to assume that nutrition will solve all GI distress. Refer for symptom management as resolution will take time, even with improved nutrition (all ED). Superior mesenteric artery syndrome is specifically caused by malnutrition and loss of adipose tissue and causes pain with eating (AN). A referral for pain management may be needed.

Vitamin D and sunlight exposure: Once thought to be a concern primarily for patients with insufficient dairy consumption or sunlight exposure, vitamin D deficiency is now recognized to be more common even in the general population.

Other Factors Associated With Insufficient Intake

Anorexia/forgetting to eat/lack of interest in food: (Note that this refers to anorexia, the symptom of poor appetite, not anorexia nervosa.) Assess sensations of appetite: Does the patient feel hungry at any time during the day? If a patient reports low or no appetite, is this a recent change?

> ***Expert Insight***
>
> *An eating disorder itself—even anorexia nervosa—does not cause poor appetite. Underlying causes may be medication side effects, depression, chronic or acute emotional distress, anxiety, limited interoceptive awareness (sometimes associated with ADHD or autism), or a medical condition, any of which should be referred to the appropriate discipline for assessment.*

Changes in appetite or taste: Loss of taste and smell is a commonly reported symptom of COVID-19. It can also result from zinc deficiency (AN, ON, ARFID), resulting in a preference for spicy foods and condiments.

> ***Expert Insight***
>
> *A recent increase in appetite not associated with a corresponding increase in physical activity should be referred for further medical assessment.*

Changes in recent food intake and recent food avoidance: Diet culture promotes the erroneous idea that intermittent fasting or "going hungry" is an effective weight-loss method. Assess for recent changes in food intake, what the patient attributes them to, and if they are getting better or worse (all ED).

Food insecurity: See Assessment of Food Availability on page 56.

Lack of strength or stamina for eating: Assess whether a patient who is acutely or chronically ill, malnourished, injured, frail, or neglected requires assistance at meals or nutrition support.

> ***Expert Insight***
>
> *Eating disorders can co-occur with any medical illness or condition. Best practice is to address malnutrition immediately, with psychiatric and psychological coordination as needed.*

Mealtime resistance or refusal to eat: Fear of eating can be a feature of all eating disorders. Even a patient who voluntarily entered treatment may struggle to eat appropriately. Assess whether a patient is able to eat independently or requires assistance at meals or nutrition support.

Nausea or early satiety: See information in Food(s) from Specific Food Groups Related to Gastrointestinal (GI) Symptoms on page 45.

Spitting food out: Chewing and spitting out food without swallowing it can be an effort to restrict caloric intake (AN), a symptom of high anxiety, or fear of choking (RD, ARFID). Assess for chewing and spitting, particularly in weight-class athletes and in individuals post-bariatric surgery.

Prolonged mealtimes: Assess for reheating food during meals, cutting and mixing foods, and other mealtime activities that abnormally lengthen mealtimes (AN, ARFID, ON). When did these routines develop? Can the patient identify a rationale? Is the behavior supportive or detrimental to their overall nutrition or functioning?

> ***Expert Insight***
>
> *If food rituals are performed in an effort to prevent something from happening or to counteract perceived contamination, a referral to a mental health provider may be appropriate, as these can be symptoms of obsessive-compulsive disorder.*

Assessment of Intake Different From Recommended

Inappropriate use of food: Diet culture, social media, incarceration, food insecurity, intergenerational history, and other factors can result in inappropriate use of food, such as food as a reward, withholding of food as a punishment, forcing children to "clean their plates" to earn dessert, and so on. Assess for food rules and practices in patients of all ages, as adults may be perpetuating behaviors linked to childhood, and teens may be learning inappropriate practices from social media (all ED).

Inappropriate choices of food (including food group and nutrient imbalance or a limited variety of food): Assess for inappropriate and unbalanced eating due to mistaken beliefs and fears about food or food insecurity (all ED).

Taking medication (over-the-counter or prescribed, including herbal, botanical, or dietary supplements that are problematic or inconsistent with recommended foods): Assess for use/abuse of over-the-counter or prescription medications, stimulants, laxatives, diet pills, and dietary supplements. Whether self-prescribed or recommended by a wellness, health, or pseudohealth professional, all such substances should be evaluated (all ED).

Expert Insight

Daily use/abuse of laxatives, stimulant medications, and prescription drugs should not be immediately discontinued except under a physician's care, as they may require a weaning protocol to prevent withdrawal symptoms.

Protein or other supplementation: Assess for excessive protein intake due to following a trendy diet, social media influencers, or as a misguided attempt to increase muscle mass or protect muscle mass during weight loss (all ED).

Assessment of Food and Nutrient Intolerance

Coughing or choking with eating: Verbally assess for the ability to chew and swallow and refer for an evaluation of swallowing impairment by a speech-language pathologist if needed.

> ***Expert Insight***
>
> *Forcible feeding by caregivers that is causing a patient to cough or choke should be immediately discontinued (ARFID).*

Diarrhea in response to high refined carbohydrate intake: Assess if this is a side-effect (BED) or a purging method (BN).

Feeling of food "getting stuck" in the throat: Assess if this is related to a past choking or anaphylactic incident, oral or esophageal condition, injury, or surgery (ARFID). Refer for an evaluation of swallowing impairment by a speech-language pathologist.

Prolonged chewing at mealtime: See Prolonged Mealtimes on page 48.

Assessment of Nutrition and Health Awareness

Awareness of food or calorie-containing beverages: Preoccupation with calorie content of food is normalized in diet culture and even in dietetics. When it becomes fear, it can impair adequate energy intake (AN, BN, BED, ON).

Avoidance of foods of age-appropriate texture: Avoiding foods due to the way they look or feel in the mouth can result in insufficient intake (ARFID). Assess for tooth or mouth pain, difficulty chewing or swallowing, and ill-fitting dentures. Refer to a speech-language pathologist as needed.

Avoidance of foods or food groups (including fear of foods or dysfunctional thoughts regarding food or food experiences): Diet culture simultaneously villainizes food and then admires the "willpower" it takes to avoid it. Ask about a patient's rationale for avoiding specific foods or food groups and assess for food restrictions that are impairing nutritional adequacy (AN, ON, ARFID). At all times encourage respect for preferences, allergies, intolerances, medical conditions, and cultural practices if nutritional adequacy can be maintained.

Belief that aging can be slowed by dietary limitations: Assess for nutritional inadequacy related to preoccupation with longevity, disease prevention, or "antiaging" products or procedures (ON).

> ***Expert Insight***
>
> *Adherents of intermittent fasting or the caloric restriction movement may cite studies "proving" that these practices extend life. Note that these studies have been performed on mice, and there is no evidence that caloric restriction can extend the human lifespan. Nevertheless, encourage respect for a patient's eating preferences if they are not impairing nutritional adequacy.*

Chronic dieting behavior (including food preoccupation and knowledge about current fad diets): Social media has expanded the reach of diet culture exponentially. Assess for nutritional adequacy and frequent changes in eating patterns due to "diet shopping" (all ED).

Cultural or religious practices that limit intake: Cultural humility prioritizes respect for cultural and religious eating practices and is a tenet in the *Code of Ethics for the Nutrition & Dietetics Profession*.[3,4] When a patient's cultural or religious practice is impairing their nutrition or harming their health or eating disorder recovery, consultation with a hospital chaplain or other representative of that faith or culture may be helpful to guide next steps (all ED).

Defensiveness, hostility, or resistance to change (including denial of hunger, denial of need for food- and nutrition-related changes, frustration or dissatisfaction with medical nutrition therapy recommendations, lack of appreciation of the importance of making recommended nutrition-related changes, unwillingness or disinterest in applying nutrition-related recommendations, verbalizing unwillingness or disinterest in learning): Patient autonomy prioritizes respect for a patient's choices and decisions and is a tenet in the *Code of Ethics for the Nutrition & Dietetics Profession*.[4,5] When an adult patient rejects nutrition recommendations or chooses to discontinue care, consult with the patient's other providers, a supervisor, or support partners to guide next steps (all ED).

Eating alone, feeling embarrassed by the amount of food eaten, eating much more rapidly than normal, eating until feeling uncomfortably full, consuming large amounts of food when not feeling hungry, feeling a sense of lack of control of overeating during the episode, and feeling disgusted with oneself, depressed, or guilty after overeating: Any eater can experience these sensations once in a while. When they are frequent, preoccupying, or impairing, they are the criteria for BED. Best practice is a mental health evaluation in addition to medical nutrition therapy (MNT).

Embarrassment or anger at need for self-monitoring and incomplete self-monitoring records: Before assigning record-keeping as an intervention, assess a patient or support partner's ability to keep records. Consider neurodiversity and options for age- and literacy-appropriate methods for gathering information.

> ### *Expert Insight*
>
> *Ask if a patient has ever kept food records and find out what they were like, how they were used, and if they have any negative connotations in the patient's experience.*

Emotional distress, anxiety, or frustration surrounding mealtimes: Ask the patient to describe their experience of eating and refer distressing emotions not related to nutrition to a mental health provider (all ED). Assess if preplanning menus, preparing a grocery list with your help, delegating meal preparation to support partners, or other changes can decrease mealtime decision-making stress. Include anyone who typically participates in meals with the patient in the planning process.

Food faddism and pica: Ingesting nonfood items to induce feelings of fullness can cause intestinal blockage and may require medical evaluation or even emergency care (AN, BN, BED). Eating clay, corn starch, or excessive quantities of ice must be evaluated in the context of cultural practices, nutritional deficiencies, and safety (P).

> ### *Expert Insight*
>
> *Habitual chewing of nonfood items such as gum, pens, drinking straws, or fingernails can be related to anxiety and may benefit from a referral to a mental health provider.*

Frustration over lack of control: A patient who is in treatment involuntarily is likely to feel frustrated over their lack of autonomy. But so is a patient who wants to change and feels ineffective or powerless to do so.

When a patient who expresses a desire to change their eating behaviors is unable to progress—even one not diagnosed with an eating disorder—a referral to a mental health provider can help with underlying emotional factors and the stress of chronic illness.

> **Expert Insight**
>
> *If frustration turns to thoughts of hopelessness and a patient indicates a wish to die, give up, or not be alive, consult immediately with the patient's other providers for direction. If you believe that a patient is in danger, contact their emergency contact or a local crisis hotline.*

Harmful beliefs and attitudes of parents and caregivers: Include support partners in your assessment as much as possible. The weight-conscious environment we live in can lead even well-meaning parents to restrict a larger child's food intake, especially if it has been recommended by a medical provider.

> **Expert Insight**
>
> *A child's illness can unsurprisingly lead a parent or caregiver to desperate measures, and unscrupulous vendors can take advantage of this desperation. Professionalism requires approaching even harmful behaviors as loving attempts to help a child, even when you are advising against them.*

Inflexibility with food selection: Patient preference for a limited variety of foods can cause nutritional inadequacy (ARFID, AN, ON). Overruling a patient's autonomy in food choices should not be undertaken lightly; only when health or functioning is impaired, or when the patient expresses a desire to expand their repertoire. If a patient's preferences, however limited, can provide for their basic nutrition needs, expansion of food selection may not be necessary (ARFID).

Irrational thoughts about food's effect on the body (weight preoccupation): Diet culture has normalized preoccupation with food's effect on body weight, but that does not make it healthy or appropriate (AN, BN, BED, PD).

Previous failures to effectively change target behavior: When a patient has tried and failed to change a behavior, best practice is to refer them to mental health care or medical evaluation for underlying issues (BN, BED, RD, PD).

Assessment of Food and Nutrient Knowledge and Skill

Limited food and nutrition-related knowledge: Even patients with extensive nutrition knowledge—including RDNs!—may not be applying it beneficially (AN, BN, BED). This is where you come in, teaching the *practice* of good nutrition, rather than simply the data.

Inability to apply food and nutrition information, inability to change food or activity behavior, inability to maintain weight or regain weight, inability or unwillingness to select food consistent with guidelines: A patient who wants to change but cannot is completely different from a patient expressing no desire to change. Consult with a supervisor or other providers to balance the importance of patient autonomy with providing appropriate care.

Impaired ability to prepare food/meals and uncertainty regarding foods to prepare based on nutrition prescription: Assess a patient's ability to self-nourish in accordance with their nutritional needs and determine what you or support partners can provide.

Assessment of Physical Activity

Decreased or sedentary activity level: Do not just assess a patient's activity level, ask about their *experience* with activity. Barriers to physical movement include bad memories of physical education, unsafe environment, joint pain, lack of suitable shoes or equipment, weight stigma, and more. In addition, inquire if a medical provider has recommended that they do not exercise.

Increased physical activity, excessive physical activity (ignoring family or job, exercising without rest days or while injured or sick), and overtraining: Excessive exercise is pathological, even dangerous, when it is out of sync with nutritional intake, used as a compensatory behavior for eating, or continued while injured (AN, BN, BED).

> ***Expert Insight***
>
> *Excessive exercise and an inability to take rest days can be a form of self-medication and may benefit from a mental health assessment for anxiety.*

Assessment of Food Availability

Economic constraints that limit availability of appropriate foods, food insecurity or unwillingness to use available resources, or inability to purchase and transport food to one's home: Economic inequity results in large groups of people who do not have enough money for food as well as areas without nearby access to grocery stores. Food insecurity is a direct risk factor for all eating disorders.[6]

Assessment of Medications and Supplements

Insulin: Insulin-dependent diabetes is a risk factor for all eating disorders as well as a specific type of compensatory behavior: under-administering insulin (or not using it at all) in order to lose weight (BN).[7-9] Symptoms include abnormal weight loss, high blood glucose levels, high HbA1c, and ketosis. Assessment for dysfunctional eating behaviors is important for all patients with diabetes, regardless of type, due to their high incidence.[9,10]

> ***Expert Insight***
>
> *"Diabulimia" is a slang term and should not be used unless preferred by a patient.*

Medication associated with weight loss, medications that cause anorexia, and medications that increase energy expenditure: Assess for medications intended to produce weight loss as well as those with weight loss or depressed appetite as a side effect (AN, BN, BED, PD). (Refer to Chapter 5 for more information on medications.)

> ***Expert Insight***
>
> *Anorexia nervosa can cause elevated serum cholesterol that will often be normalized with nutritional rehabilitation.*[9]

Medication (lipid lowering): Assess for use, refusal, or withholding of lipid-lowering medication by a medical provider.[11]

Medications associated with increased appetite, medications that affect appetite, medications that affect resting metabolic rate, medications that impair fluid excretion, and medications that reduce requirements or impair metabolism: Assess for medications intended to produce weight gain as well as those with weight gain or increased appetite as a side effect. Assess medication compliance, as a patient may be reluctant to take a prescribed medication due to fear of weight gain (AN, BN, BED, PD).

Medications requiring nutrient supplementation that cannot be accomplished with food intake and medications with known food-medication interactions: Assess for compliance with medication-related eating instructions, as a patient with an eating disorder may have difficulty eating or not eating with medication as prescribed (AN, BN, BED, PD).

Expert Insight

Any use of ipecac syrup should be immediately reported to the medical provider.

Expert Insight

Assess whether the patient is vomiting after taking their medication, in which case they may not be retaining the active ingredients.

Misuse of laxatives, enemas, diuretics, stimulants, and metabolic enhancers: Assess for compensatory behaviors using over-the-counter or prescription medications (BN).

Nutrition Assessment: Biochemical Data, Medical Tests, and Procedures

Blood tests: When assessing biochemical data, it is crucial to recognize that even severely dysfunctional eating can produce normal-seeming laboratory values.[12] Patients, support partners, and other health care providers may take normal results at face value, using them to deny existence of a problem. They are not considering that dehydration can conceal deficiencies, long-term malnutrition causes metabolic and behavioral changes that conserve nutrient use, circulating nutrient levels can be within normal limits even when nutrient stores are severely depleted,

> ***Expert Insight***
>
> *Always consider test results in context with other factors rather than as standalone measures.*

and intake of micronutrient supplements or fortified foods can mask nutritional deficiencies. By the time blood test results have progressed to abnormal levels, deficiencies are serious and potentially life-threatening. Blood tests related to eating disorders are summarized in Box 3.2 on page 60.

Bone density testing: The results of a dual-energy x-ray absorptiometry scan (DEXA or DXA) describe a person's bone mineral density compared with an age- and sex-matched control group. Osteopenia, osteoporosis, and "stress" fractures result from dysfunctional eating and hormonal

BOX 3.2 Blood Tests Related to Eating Disorders

Albumin

Relationship to eating disorders

No longer considered a reliable indicator of nutrition status

Amylase

Relationship to eating disorders

Digestive enzyme produced mainly in salivary glands and pancreas. Inflammation due to self-induced vomiting may allow salivary isoamylase into the bloodstream, but serum amylase can also be caused by binge eating, even in the absence of vomiting; that is, elevated amylase should not be assumed to be evidence of purging

May be elevated due to

Binge eating (bulimia nervosa [BN], binge-eating disorder [BED])[a]

Induced vomiting (BN, purging disorder [PD], rumination disorder [RD])

Cholecystitis (gallbladder infection)

Infection or obstruction of salivary glands (BN, PD)

Intestinal obstruction (pica)

Pancreatic or bile duct obstruction

Perforated ulcer

Tubal pregnancy (may be ruptured)

Viral gastroenteritis

Macroamylasemia

May be decreased due to

Low carbohydrate intake

Damage to the pancreas

Kidney disease

Pancreatic cancer

Toxemia of pregnancy

Nutrition Assessment

BOX 3.2 Blood Tests Related to Eating Disorders(cont.)

Blood urea nitrogen (BUN)

Relationship to eating disorders

Evaluates kidney function, which can be compromised any time nutrition is insufficient, regardless of current body weight

May be elevated due to

Dehydration (All eating disorders [ED])

Muscle-wasting/catabolism of somatic protein/starvation (anorexia nervosa [AN], orthorexia nervosa [ON], avoidant/restrictive food intake disorder [ARFID])

Excessive dietary protein intake (ON)

Impaired kidney function

Decreased blood flow to the kidneys due to congestive heart failure, shock, stress, recent heart attack, or severe burns

Obstructed urine flow

May be decreased due to

Starvation (AN, ON, ARFID)

Overhydration

Liver disease

Calcium

Relationship to eating disorders

Note: Serum calcium level is not a direct reflection of dietary calcium intake

May be elevated due to

Hyperparathyroidism

Bone cancer

May be decreased due to

Malnutrition (all ED)

Alcoholism

Magnesium deficiency (all ED)

Vitamin D deficiency (all ED)

Hypoparathyroidism

Continued on next page

BOX 3.2 Blood Tests Related to Eating Disorders (cont.)

Complement C3

Relationship to eating disorders

Sensitive indicator of nutrition status

May be elevated due to

Cancer

Ulcerative colitis

May be decreased due to

Malnutrition (all ED)

Cirrhosis

Hepatitis

Lupus

Creatinine (sCR)

Relationship to eating disorders

Evaluates kidney function, which can be compromised any time nutrition is insufficient, regardless of current body weight

May be elevated due to

Dehydration (all ED)

Muscle injury

Kidney stone

Substance abuse

Urinary tract obstruction

Decreased blood flow to the kidneys due to shock, congestive heart failure, atherosclerosis, or complications of diabetes

May be decreased due to

Muscle wasting (all ED)

Pregnancy (due to increased blood volume)

BOX 3.2 Blood Tests Related to Eating Disorders (cont.)

Ferritin

Relationship to eating disorders

Most sensitive indicator of iron status

May be elevated due to

Excessive iron supplementation (ON)

Inflammation

Liver disease

Hemochromatosis (iron storage disease)

May be decreased due to

Insufficient dietary intake of iron (all ED)

Folate (vitamin B9)

Relationship to eating disorders

Indicator of nutrition status; deficiency can cause altered mental status

May be elevated due to

Pernicious anemia

Liver dysfunction

May be decreased due to

Malnutrition (all ED)

Alcohol abuse

Celiac disease (AN, ON, ARFID)

Crohn's disease

Hemolytic anemia

Glucose

Relationship to eating disorders

Indicator of bloodstream energy supply

May be elevated due to

Type 2 diabetes (all ED)

Type 1 diabetes secondary to insufficient insulin (all ED)

Continued on next page

BOX 3.2 Blood Tests Related to Eating Disorders (cont.)

Glucose (cont.)

May be decreased due to

Acute malnutrition/fasting (all ED)

Insufficient carbohydrate intake (all ED)

Excess insulin administration

Hematocrit

Relationship to eating disorders

Indicator of nutrition status

May be elevated due to

Dehydration (all ED)

Polycythemia (blood disorder)

Blood doping

Anabolic steroid use

May be decreased due to

Malnutrition (all ED)

Insufficient dietary intake of iron (all ED)

Hemoglobin

Relationship to eating disorders

Indicator of nutrition status

May be elevated due to

Dehydration (all ED)

May be decreased due to

Malnutrition (all ED)

Insufficient dietary intake of iron (all ED)

Human chorionic gonadotropin (hCG)

Relationship to eating disorders

Indicator of pregnancy

BOX 3.2 Blood Tests Related to Eating Disorders(cont.)

Human chorionic gonadotropin (cont.)

May be elevated due to

Pregnancy

Note: hCG injections (those touted as a weight-loss method but not US Food and Drug Administration [FDA]-approved for weight loss) will not cause a positive pregnancy test

Iron

Relationship to eating disorders

Indicator of nutrition status; deficiency can cause headache and fatigue, difficulty concentrating

May be elevated due to

Excessive iron supplementation (ON)

Hemochromatosis

May be decreased due to

Insufficient dietary intake of iron (all ED)

Vegetarian, vegan, or plant-based dietary pattern (AN, ON, ARFID)

Heavy or long duration of menstruation

Pregnancy

Rapid growth in children

Lipase

Relationship to eating disorders

Indicator of pancreas function affected by fluctuating eating behaviors

May be elevated due to

Pancreatitis (AN, BN)

Kidney disease

Salivary gland inflammation (BN, PD)

Bowel obstruction (Pica)

Peptic ulcer

May be decreased due to

Permanent pancreas damage

Continued on next page

BOX 3.2 Blood Tests Related to Eating Disorders (cont.)

Liver function tests: alanine transaminase (ALT), alkaline phosphatase (ALP), aspartate transaminase (AST)

Relationship to eating disorders

Evaluate liver function, which can be compromised by ED

May be elevated due to

Substance abuse (includes drugs, alcohol, and steroids)

Malnutrition (all ED)

Hepatitis

Magnesium

Relationship to eating disorders

Indicator of kidney and gastrointestinal function

May be elevated due to

Dehydration (all ED)

Laxative abuse (BN, PD) if contain magnesium

Excessive use of over-the-counter antacids containing magnesium

Hypothyroidism

Addison disease

May be decreased due to

Insufficient dietary intake of magnesium (all ED)

Diuretic abuse (all ED)

Laxative abuse (BN, PD)

Alcohol abuse

Hypoparathyroidism

Crohn's disease

Irritable bowel disease (AN, ON, ARFID)

Celiac disease (AN, ON, ARFID)

Surgery

Burns

Pregnancy

BOX 3.2 Blood Tests Related to Eating Disorders(cont.)

Mean corpuscular volume (MCV)

Relationship to eating disorders

Indicator of nutrition status

May be elevated due to

Vitamin B12 deficiency (macrocytic/megaloblastic) anemia (all ED)

Alcoholism

May be decreased due to

Iron deficiency (microcytic) anemia (all ED)

Thalassemia

Phosphorus

Relationship to eating disorders

Indicator of nutrition status

May be elevated due to

Excessive supplementation of phosphorous

May be decreased due to

Refeeding syndrome (AN, ON)

Vomiting (BN, PD)

Laxative abuse (BN, PD)

Diuretic abuse (all ED)

Alcohol abuse

Thyroid disease

Type 2 diabetes

Kidney disease

Malabsorption

Potassium

Relationship to eating disorders

Indicator of nutrition status

Continued on next page

BOX 3.2 Blood Tests Related to Eating Disorders (cont.)

Potassium (cont.)

May be elevated due to

Dehydration due to insufficient fluid intake (all ED)

Type 2 diabetes

Kidney disease

Excessive supplementation of potassium or intake of foods high in potassium (ON)

Tissue injury, burns

Addison disease

Hypoaldosteronism

Overuse of nonsteroidal anti-inflammatory drugs (NSAIDs), beta blockers, angiotensin-converting enzyme (ACE) inhibitors, and potassium-sparing diuretics

May be decreased due to

Refeeding syndrome (AN, ON)

Malnutrition (all ED)

Vomiting (BN, PD)

Dehydration due to diarrhea (BN, PD)

Acetaminophen overdose

Hyperaldosteronism

Abuse of diuretics (all ED)

Corticosteroids, alpha- and beta-adrenergic agonists, gentamicin, carbenicillin, amphotericin B, even when used as recommended

Red blood cell count (RBC)

Relationship to eating disorders

Indicator of nutrition status

May be elevated due to

Dehydration (all ED)

May be decreased due to

Iron deficiency (all ED)

BOX 3.2 Blood Tests Related to Eating Disorders(cont.)

Thyroid-stimulating hormone (TSH)

Relationship to eating disorders

Indicator of thyroid function. Note: abnormal thyroid function impacts appetite and weight and can both predate and result from ED

May be elevated due to

Starvation (AN, ON, ARFID)

Hypothyroidism (acute or chronic)

Pituitary tumor

Insufficient administration of prescribed thyroid hormone

May be decreased due to

Hyperthyroidism

Excessive administration of prescribed thyroid hormone (AN, BN, BED)

Damage to the pituitary gland

Total protein

Relationship to eating disorders

Indicator of nutrition status

May be elevated due to

Chronic infections

HIV

May be decreased due to

Insufficient dietary intake of protein (all ED)

Celiac disease (AN, ON, ARFID)

Irritable bowel disease (AN, ON, ARFID)

Kidney disease

Liver disease

Continued on next page

BOX 3.2 Blood Tests Related to Eating Disorders (cont.)

Vitamin B12

Relationship to eating disorders

Indicator of nutrition status; deficiency can cause altered mental status, contribute to depression

May be elevated due to

Serious underlying illness such as liver disease, kidney failure, leukemia, polycythemia vera, hypereosinophilic syndrome

May be decreased due to

Vitamin B12 intake deficiency (pernicious) anemia (AN, ON, ARFID)

Vegetarian, vegan, or plant-based dietary pattern (AN, ON, ARFID)

Post-bariatric surgery, especially Roux-en-Y gastric bypass, due to loss of intrinsic factor secreted in stomach

Zinc

Relationship to eating disorders

Indicator of nutrition status; deficiency can cause altered sense of taste, difficulty gaining weight, and symptoms of depression

May be elevated due to

Excessive zinc supplementation (ON)

May be decreased due to

Malnutrition (all ED)

Vegetarian, vegan, or plant-based dietary pattern (AN, ON, ARFID)

High alcohol intake

Chronic diarrhea (BN, PD)

Excessive exercise (all ED)

Sickle cell disease

Chronic liver disease

Post-bariatric surgery (all ED)

BOX 3.2 Blood Tests Related to Eating Disorders(cont.)

25-hydroxyvitamin D

Relationship to eating disorders

Vitamin D deficiency can cause depression and inability to reverse bone loss

May be elevated due to

Excessive vitamin D supplementation (ON)

May be decreased due to

Insufficient vitamin D intake (all ED)

Insufficient fatty acid intake (all ED)

Lack of exposure to sunlight

Malabsorption

Liver and kidney diseases

Some medications, including phenytoin, phenobarbital, and rifampin, even when used as prescribed

[a] Abbreviations in parentheses indicate suggested eating disorders to screen for.

Expert Insight

A patient restricted from exercise may incorrectly believe they need to decrease their energy intake to compensate for less physical activity.

deficiencies that impair bone metabolism, and although medication may be prescribed, the most effective known treatment is weight restoration through MNT.[13] Restrictions on physical activity due to bone fracture risk range from not participating in athletics to using a wheelchair and even bed rest.

Electrocardiogram (EKG or ECG) and echocardiogram (echo): Results may show damage to heart muscle and function that can result from

> ***Expert Insight***
>
> *Any patient who has rapidly lost weight or has lost a significant percentage of body weight should be evaluated for cardiac stability regardless of their current weight or diagnosis.*

dysfunctional eating. These may be asymptomatic ("silent") or experienced by the patient as heart pounding or missed heartbeats, shortness of breath, chest pain at rest or during exercise, general weakness, dizziness upon standing, or edema. Intervention may include physical activity restrictions including wheelchair use or bed rest, or ongoing cardiac monitoring.

Urinary tests: Urine output and urine specific gravity (USG) are indicators of an individual's hydration status. Urine output fluctuates daily based on recent fluid and sodium intake, while USG is a more sensitive measure of fluid balance. Elevated USG results from dehydration due to insufficient fluid intake (AN, ON, ARFID) or diarrhea (BN, PD), urinary tract infection, and excess sweating. Low USG may indicate excessive fluid intake (all ED) and also occurs in kidney failure and diabetes insipidus.

Nutrition Assessment: Anthropometric Measurements

Standalone anthropometric measurements that attempt to measure weight or body composition have limited use in eating disorder assessment. To be effective as a data point, a patient's current weight or body composition must be considered within the context of changes over time, overall growth and development, health, and specific conditions (both acute and chronic), injuries, disabilities, and so on.

To place a patient's current weight in context requires a pediatric growth chart if available; a weight history including usual, highest, and lowest adult weights, if known; degree of weight change as a percentage of previous weight; and time frame of that weight change. This information can be gathered from the patient, support partners, other providers, and the medical record.

Acute weight change is significant for malnutrition, as are repeated fluctuations and failure to follow an expected growth curve for either weight or height. When long-term data is not available, or in emergency situations, vital signs can be used as a proxy for acute nutrition and hydration status. Frequent remeasuring of weight is not useful unless input and output are also being measured.

The harm caused by inappropriate focus on weight and BMI in eating disorder care cannot be overstated. Weight and body composition methods that depend on weight are specifically inappropriate for eating disorder assessment, not least of all because harmful weight loss and weight loss practices do not always result in the individual being underweight. Other harms of using weight and body composition in eating disorder care include[14]:

- They do not accurately measure malnutrition or other underlying processes.
- Weight and size standards are based on populations, not individuals.
- Standards do not account for diversity of gender or race, therefore individuals of mixed heritage or from marginalized groups will be compared to standards that do not apply to them.
- Acute illness status leads to inaccuracies because the standards are based on a generally well population.
- They reflect long-term nutrition status rather than acute illness.
- Results vary depending on hydration status—a problem in itself—but this also means they can be manipulated.
- Measurement errors occur more often in fat individuals.
- "Normal" results can provide false reassurance.

The process of being weighed and measured can be distressing and should be performed in a trauma-informed manner with the intention of maintaining patient safety at all times.[15] For example:

- Ask for permission to weigh the patient and respect their choice not to be weighed.

- If the patient consents to be weighed, ask for and honor their preferences on any of the following options that are permitted:
  - to weigh at the beginning or end of the appointment;
  - to face the scale or away from it;
  - to know their weight or not;
  - to wear their clothes or change into a gown.
- If the patient requests that they not be shown their weight, do not document it in a place the patient can access.
- Treat weight like any other vital sign: a neutral piece of information about a natural bodily function. Refrain from commenting on the patient's current weight or weight change. "Better" or "Good job!" may not mean the same thing to the patient as it does to you.
- Under no circumstances should you ever comment on your own weight in front of a patient.

For further discussion of body weight related to eating disorder care, refer to the Weight section in Chapter 6, Nutrition Intervention for Eating Disorders: Nutrition Education.

Nutrition Assessment: Nutrition Focused Physical Findings

Visible symptoms of dysfunctional eating behaviors vary from person to person and range from neutral to life-threatening. Although any information gathered through a nutrition focused physical examination (NFPE) should be documented, be aware that—as with laboratory values and anthropometrics—an individual can be severely ill, malnourished,

Expert Insight

Trauma-informed care includes asking for permission before examining an individual.

BOX 3.3 Nutrition Focused Physical Findings Related to Eating Disorders

Head and neck

Ketone smell on breath indicates insufficient carbohydrate intake (anorexia nervosa [AN], orthorexia nervosa [ON])[a]

Mouth sores can be caused by vomiting (bulimia nervosa [BN], purging disorder [PD])

Dry or cracked lips suggest vitamin deficiency or dehydration[b] (all eating disorders [ED])

Enlarged/inflamed parotid glands in the neck from frequent vomiting[b] (BN, PD)

Damaged or missing teeth due to erosion by stomach acid during vomiting[b] (BN, PD)

Hair loss due to malnutrition[b] (all ED)

Lanugo (fine hair) on face due to malnutrition, low body temperature[b] (all ED)

Palate abrasions caused by finger or foreign object to induce vomiting (BN, PD)

Broken blood vessel in eye due to vomiting[b] (BN, PD)

Eyes appear sunken due to muscle wasting and loss of visible orbital fat pads beneath the eyes[b] (all ED)

Dark circles beneath eyes[b] (all ED)

Torso, front and back

Abdominal distension after eating

Ribs and depressions between ribs visible through skin on back

Iliac crest (hipbone) visibly protruding

Prominently protruding clavicle[b]

Prominently protruding acromion bone (where clavicle meets shoulder)

Prominent kneecap when leg is bent

Limbs and extremities

Acrocyanosis of hands and feet caused by malnutrition, low body temperature, or reduced cardiac function (AN, ON)

Delayed capillary refill rate[b] (when a patient clenches and then opens their fist, or crosses then uncrosses their legs, palm or leg stays white while capillaries refill with blood) (all ED)

Russell sign (scars, scabs on knuckles) from using fingers to induce vomiting (BN, PD)

Fluid accumulation at ankles, pitting edema due to malnutrition (all ED)

Continued on next page

BOX 3.3 Nutrition Focused Physical Findings Related to Eating Disorders (cont.)

Skin

Dry skin due to malnutrition (all ED)

Acanthosis nigricans (dark ring of skin around neck) suggests insulin resistance (binge-eating disorder [BED])

Vital signs (all ED)

Each of the following suggest metabolic conservation effects of starvation:

- low blood pressure
- drop in blood pressure upon standing
- low heart rate
- dizziness upon standing or walking across a room[b]
- decreased temperature

Other

Visible blood in emesis due to esophageal erosion or broken blood vessels from repeated vomiting (BN, PD)

Visible blood in stool due to constipation leading to hemorrhoids, misuse of laxatives (BN, PD)

[a] Abbreviations in parentheses denote specific eating disorders that may be indicated.
[b] Signs that may be visible during a video session.

or both, and not exhibit any of these signs. Box 3.3 lists nutrition focused physical findings associated with eating disorders.

Ethical dietetics practice requires us not to mistake the appearance of "normal" or "above normal" weight as a proxy for health or nutritional stability. The information in Box 3.3 should be used as a guide, not a diagnostic tool, and a lack of physical findings should not be equated with satisfactory nutrition status.

> ***Expert Insight***
>
> *While gathering this information, an RDN may learn about psychological, social, and emotional issues that cannot be resolved with MNT. Chapter 8 provides guidance on referral to mental health care.*

Nutrition Assessment: Client History

An individual's combined medical and social history contributes to the full picture of their nutrition status and informs the nutrition diagnosis and treatment plan. The following sections detail areas to consider, with suggestions in parentheses for eating disorders that may be related.

Social History

Physical, emotional, or sexual abuse: Tragically, information on the intersection of abuse and eating dysfunction could fill a library. When any kind of abuse or trauma is suspected or reported, follow facility protocol and communicate with the patient's mental health professional and with a supervisor.

Avoidance of social events where food is served: Individuals with eating disorders may avoid social eating situations due to dislike of the sounds of others chewing (ARFID), fear of losing control (BED, BN), discomfort with being observed while eating (all ED), history of weight-related bullying (all ED), history of being criticized for food selectivity (ARFID, ON), uncertainty about what food may be served and how to make selections that meet dietary needs, fear of contact with a known allergen, or an underlying anxiety disorder.

Change in living environment and independence: Transitions are stressful and can impact eating, even if they are wanted and perceived as positive. Increasing independence can highlight an individual's lack of experience in obtaining and preparing food and can provide opportunities for more secretive behaviors (all ED). Decreasing independence, for example due to aging or injury, or as experienced during the COVID-19 lock down period, can exacerbate existing eating issues or create new ones (all ED).

Substance abuse: Substances of abuse can include over-the-counter laxatives, diuretics, diet pills, ergogenic aids, and stimulants in addition to street drugs, prescription drugs, and anabolic steroids (all ED). Note: Any patient reporting current or past use of ipecac syrup should be instructed to stop immediately and be referred for cardiac evaluation.

Lack of developmental readiness: Neurodivergence, pervasive developmental delay, or disability may impact an individual's abilities to obtain and prepare food and to eat independently (all ED).

Lack of funds for purchase of appropriate foods: Food insecurity and poverty are direct risk factors for dysfunctional eating behavior (all ED).

Lack of suitable support system to access food: Children and teenagers without income or transportation and adults with physical or intellectual disabilities may rely on others to obtain and prepare their food. Dysfunctional eating behaviors can result if assistance is unavailable or unreliable (all ED).

Recent lifestyle changes: When transitions are overwhelming, stress hormones can influence appetite, while diet culture can propose weight loss as a method of "taking control" of a situation. Dieting does not solve the situation, but it can lead to an eating disorder.

New medical diagnosis or change in condition: A new diagnosis, especially one that requires a special diet or change in eating habits, is a known trigger for dysfunctional eating. For someone with an existing eating disorder, a new diagnosis or change in condition can be especially challenging to their recovery.

Personal and Family History

History of childhood obesity/history of familial obesity: Being labeled "obese" in childhood strongly affects a person's self-concept. If family members chronically diet or exhibit other dysfunctional eating behaviors, a child may not have any role models for internally guided eating. Weight loss efforts begun in childhood can have lifelong destructive effects, including development of eating disorders (AN, BN, BED, PD).

History of eating disorder, depression, obsessive compulsive disorders, or anxiety disorders: Although the genetic mechanism is not known,

> ***Expert Insight***
>
> *Hormone abnormalities often go undiagnosed when they are disguised by dysfunctional eating or labeled as "weight problems." Undiagnosed diabetes, polycystic ovary syndrome (PCOS), hyper- and hypothyroidism, Cushing syndrome, and others can all interfere with appetite and body weight regulation. If a patient describes a mismatch between eating and weight, such as gaining weight while dieting, unintentional dramatic weight change without a change in eating, or unexplained change in appetite, referral for an endocrine evaluation is appropriate.*

family psychiatric history, including history of alcoholism or addiction, is a risk factor for eating disorder development (all ED).

History of hyperlipidemia, atherosclerosis, or pancreatitis: Family history of heart disease is a known risk factor for dysfunctional eating when it results in excessive restriction or preoccupation with food content and quality (ON, AN).

History of inability to lose weight through conventional intervention: Focus on weight loss and frustration with weight loss attempts can lead to desperation and harmful behaviors (AN, BN, BED).

Medical and Health History

Alcoholism: Although the mechanism is not known, there appears to be a genetic link between alcohol dependence and eating disorders, with a significant co-occurrence rate with BN.

Anxiety disorder: There are many connections between anxiety and eating disorders. Anxiety about eating and after eating is a hallmark feature of most eating disorders (AN, ON, BN, BED, ARFID, PD). Sometimes dysfunctional eating behaviors develop as a form of self-medication for generalized or social anxiety, and the process of eating recovery can provoke more anxiety.

Binge eating: Binge eating is a diagnostic of BED and BN, but it can also occur as part of AN, ARFID, ON, and PD.

Cardiovascular disease, hyperlipidemia, hypertriglyceridemia, hypertension, and metabolic syndrome: A diagnosis of cardiovascular disease or one or more risk factors delivered with recommendations for dietary changes or weight loss that may not be appropriate or take into account a patient's current eating disorder status can lead to harmful eating behaviors.

Celiac disease, Crohn's disease, diverticulitis, gastroesophageal reflux disease, inflammatory bowel disease, irritable bowel syndrome, lactase deficiency, malabsorption, maldigestion, polyps in the colon, and prolapsing hemorrhoids: Any painful gastrointestinal condition, or one that requires dietary modification, can lead to dysfunctional eating behaviors in an attempt to manage symptoms or find a cure for an undiagnosed problem (AN, ON, ARFID).

Chronic fatigue syndrome/myalgic encephalomyelitis (CFS/ME): Individuals with CFS/ME may have difficulty performing food procurement and preparation tasks. AN may also increase the risk of developing CFS/ME, but the mechanism of action is unknown.

Cleft lip or palate and oral soft tissue infection: Any condition of the mouth can result in oral aversion and impact oral intake (ARFID).

Concussion: Traumatic brain injury can impact appetite, mood, and other aspects of personality and self-regulation.

Constipation: Constipation can predate dysfunctional eating behaviors or be a result of them (AN, ARFID). Fad diets low in fiber can cause constipation. Discomfort can cause reluctance to eat as well as attempts to self-medicate with laxatives, which over time can lead to dependence or abuse (BN).

Cushing syndrome: A primary symptom is weight gain, which can trigger, or be mistaken for, dysfunctional eating or dieting behavior.

Cystic fibrosis, diabetes: Both conditions require dietary modification as well as disruption to activities of daily life. Chronic stress and the required extra focus on food and eating, along with medications that may cause weight gain, are risk factors for eating dysfunction (all ED).

Dementia: As dementia progresses, cooking can become unsafe, an individual may forget to eat and ultimately may not be able to self-nourish.

Depression: Depression commonly co-occurs with all eating disorder types, both as a preexisting condition and as a result of inadequate nutrition. The long-term nature of eating disorder treatment and setbacks can add to feelings of depression and hopelessness. Suicide is a leading cause of death in individuals with eating disorders.

Fatigue: Chronic fatigue can be a result of malnutrition or of a different underlying condition and can impair the individual's ability to obtain and prepare food.

Foodborne illness: Aversion to certain foods or all foods can be the result of a distressing encounter with or reaction to eating.

Fractures (stress): Stress or overuse fractures are a key feature of relative energy deficiency in sport (REDs) that can accompany AN.

Headache: Can result from both malnutrition and dehydration (AN, BN, PD, ARFID, ON).

Hyperthyroidism, hypothyroidism, hypoglycemia: Malnutrition disrupts endocrine function, and endocrine dysfunction disrupts appetite. Hypothyroidism and hypoglycemia may resolve with nutrition rehabilitation, or they may become chronic conditions (AN, BN, BED).

Illness (Recent): In diet culture, involuntary weight loss caused by an illness can lead to harmful weight control practices to prevent weight restoration. In cases where a long-term illness leads to job loss or isolation, social and economic factors can influence eating (AN, ON).

Mental illness: Eating disorders co-occur frequently with other psychiatric conditions. Some medications for these conditions have dramatic appetite and weight-related side effects.

> ***Expert Insight***
>
> *Consult with a patient's mental health provider for assistance in learning about their diagnosis and to collaborate in the patient's care.*

Multiple sclerosis: A life-changing, chronic condition that can contribute to depression and affect an individual's mobility and ability for self-care.

Obesity and overweight: These problematic labels both contribute to and mask eating disorders for individuals whose bodies do not fit within diet culture standards.

Personality disorder: Personality disorders are not well-understood, but when present they can complicate eating disorder recovery.

Polycystic ovary disease: Because this condition can result in weight gain, weight loss is often incorrectly and ineffectively prescribed. Without accurate diagnosis and treatment, dysfunctional eating behaviors may result (BN, BED, AN).

Premenstrual syndrome: As with any condition that causes abdominal distension or discomfort, premenstrual and menstrual hormonal shifts can trigger dysfunctional eating behaviors in attempt to find relief.

Tardive dyskinesia: Involuntary movements result from certain antipsychotic medications. Depending on what part of the body is affected, tardive dyskinesia can interfere with eating ability and can increase energy needs.

Tremors: Tremors, whether due to alcohol withdrawal or any other factor, can interfere with eating ability.

Other Issues

Abdominal cramping, abdominal pain, bloating, constipation, diarrhea, epigastric pain, flatulence, gastrointestinal disturbances, nausea, and self-induced vomiting: As noted earlier, anything that causes abdominal pain or discomfort can impair eating and lead to harmful behaviors. Although gastrointestinal distress is common after long periods of starvation or vomiting, they may not resolve with nutritional rehabilitation. Medical evaluation and symptom management may be appropriate.

Amenorrhea: Historically, menstrual status was a diagnostic criteria for AN. Now it is considered simply one of many possible symptoms of malnutrition and should not be used to rule in or rule out an eating disorder.

Anorexia: A lack of appetite can be caused by a variety of factors, including certain medications, medical conditions, and depression. It is incorrect to assume that an individual with AN does not experience hunger.

Dizziness and unexplained falls, muscle weakness, fatigue, cardiac arrhythmia, dehydration, electrolyte imbalance, and shortness of breath: Inadequate nutrition and dehydration can impair balance and cause dizziness and falls. Arrhythmia and electrolyte imbalance are dangerous. Seek medical consultation if any of these are reported.

Report of always feeling cold: Cold intolerance is a physiological adaptation to starvation; body temperature decreases and adipose tissue normally used to produce heat and insulate the core is used for energy.

Medical Treatments or Procedures

Chemotherapy with oral side effects, radiation therapy, or surgery: Cancer as a life-altering diagnosis, cancer treatment and medications, and weight gain related to treatment can all impact appetite and eating behaviors. Cancer in an area that impacts eating, digestion, or elimination potentially multiplies this effect.

Bariatric surgery: Any gastrointestinal surgery should be considered a risk factor for eating disorder development. Gastrointestinal surgery also intended to cause malnutrition should be expected to also cause dysfunctional eating behavior.

Knee surgery: Knee injury is one of the most common athletic career-ending injuries. Athletes at the competitive and elite levels have dedicated much or most of their lives to their sport, and being unable to compete can be devastating to their identity and self-esteem. Patients in this situation require nutrition counseling regarding their nutrient and energy needs for healing and then on an ongoing basis if their level of physical activity will be drastically different post surgery.

Oral surgery: Oral surgery can impair the ability and desire to eat and may cause pain with chewing, swallowing, or both. Involuntary weight loss caused by an inability to eat normally can trigger an eating disorder.

Ostomy: An ostomy can result from laxative abuse and further reduce willingness to eat (AN, BN).

These lists, while extensive, do not include every individual factor that could contribute to an eating disorder or be noted in a nutrition assessment. Identifying the pieces of each individual's eating situation can be an ongoing process that occurs over time. The initial assessment will inform the initial nutrition diagnosis, with the option to revise and update as needed.

References

1. Academy of Nutrition and Dietetics. NCP Step 1: Nutrition Assessment. eNCPT website. 2023. Accessed June 25, 2024. www.ncpro.org//pubs/2023-encpt-en/category-1
2. Academy of Nutrition and Dietetics. Nutrition Assessment and Monitoring and Evaluation Terminology. eNCPT website. 2023. Accessed June 25, 2024. www.ncpro.org/pubs/2023-encpt-en/page-006
3. Palmer S. Cultural humility in food & nutrition. *Today's Dietitian*. 2021;23(2). Accessed June 26, 2024. www.todaysdietitian.com/newarchives/0221p24.shtml
4. Academy of Nutrition and Dietetics. Code of Ethics for the Nutrition & Dietetics Profession. eatrightPRO website. 2018. Accessed June 26, 2024. www.eatrightpro.org/practice/code-of-ethics/code-of-ethics-for-the-nutrition-and-dietetics-profession
5. Fornari A. Approaches to ethical decision-making. *J Acad Nutr Diet*. 2015;115(1):119-121. doi:10.1016/j.jand.2014.10.026
6. Hazzard VM, Loth KA, Hooper L, Becker CB. Food insecurity and eating disorders: a review of emerging evidence. *Curr Psychiatry Rep*. 2020;22(12):74. doi:10.1007/s11920-020-01200-0
7. Mathieu J. What is diabulimia? *J Am Diet Assoc*. 2008;108(5):769-770. doi:10.1016/j.jada.2008.03.031
8. Torjesen I. Diabulimia: the world's most dangerous eating disorder. *BMJ*. 2019;364:l982. doi:10.1136/bmj.l982
9. Goebel-Fabbri AE, Fikkan J, Franko DL, Pearson K, Anderson BJ, Weinger K. Insulin restriction and associated morbidity and mortality in women with type 1 diabetes. *Diabetes Care*. 2008;31(3):415-419. doi:10.2337/dc07-2026
10. Nicolau J, Simó R, Sanchís P, et al. Eating disorders are frequent among type 2 diabetic patients and are associated with worse metabolic and psychological outcomes: results from a cross-sectional study in primary and secondary care settings. *Acta Diabetol*. 2015;52(6):1037-1044. doi:10.1007/s00592-015-0742-z

11. Rigaud D, Tallonneau I, Vergès B. Hypercholesterolaemia in anorexia nervosa: frequency and changes during refeeding. *Diabetes Metab.* 2009;35(1):57-63. doi:10.1016/j.diabet.2008.08.004
12. Setnick J. Micronutrient deficiencies and supplementation in anorexia and bulimia nervosa: a review of literature. *Nutr Clin Pract.* 2010;25(2):137-142. doi:10.1177/0884533610361478
13. Steinman J, Shibli-Rahhal A. Anorexia nervosa and osteoporosis: pathophysiology and treatment. *J Bone Metab.* 2019;26(3):133-143. doi:10.11005/jbm.2019.26.3.133
14. Casadei K, Kiel J. *Anthropometric Measurement.* StatPearls; 2022. September 26, 2022. Accessed June 26, 2024. www.ncbi.nlm.nih.gov/books/NBK537315/
15. Froreich FV, Ratcliffe SE, Vartanian LR. Blind versus open weighing from an eating disorder patient perspective. *J Eat Disord.* 2020;8:39. doi:10.1186/s40337-020-00316-1

CHAPTER 4

Nutrition Diagnosis for Eating Disorders

Nutrition diagnosis is the part of the Nutrition Care Process that specifies the main problem(s) a registered dietitian nutritionist (RDN) is going to address for a specific individual in their care.[1] This is different from the eating disorder diagnosis and is given even if the patient does not have an eating disorder diagnosis from a mental health professional or meet the *Diagnostic and Statistical Manual of Mental Disorders, 5th Edition, Text Revision* (*DSM-5-TR*) eating disorder criteria.

In fact, nutrition diagnoses free RDNs from the limitations of the *DSM-5-TR* and allow us to create a targeted, individualized description of an individual's experience. We have no need to distinguish between anorexia nervosa and atypical anorexia nervosa; bulimia nervosa and bulimia nervosa of low frequency or limited duration; or binge-eating disorder and binge-eating disorder of low frequency or limited duration, as the eating behaviors and nutrition-related goals are the same.

When an individual is experiencing dysfunctional eating behaviors, there are usually multiple nutrition-related issues for the RDN to address. For purposes of a nutrition diagnosis statement, the most pertinent and urgent nutrition diagnosis should be used.

Nutrition diagnoses are generally written in PES (problem, etiology, signs and symptoms) format:

[Nutrition diagnosis term (problem)] related to [etiology] as evidenced by [signs and symptoms].

The most important facet of a nutrition diagnosis is that it is individualized to the greatest need of each patient. It then serves as a summary to inform the next steps in the Nutrition Care Process. The examples below are sample nutrition diagnoses that may be applicable to different types of dysfunctional eating behaviors. Of course, they do not cover every possibility but can be used as a guide.

- Inadequate energy intake related to recent bereavement resulting in lack of appetite/interest in food, as evidenced by patient report of going one or more days without eating two to three times per week, dizziness upon standing, and 3% weight loss in 2 weeks.
- Inadequate energy intake related to anxiety, as evidenced by stated fear of food and incorrect beliefs about the effects of food on the body.
- Inadequate energy intake related to history of food insecurity, as evidenced by hoarding of food in the home and rationing of food throughout the month.
- Inadequate energy intake related to avoidant/restrictive food intake disorder (ARFID) as evidenced by preference for warm foods and patient having moved to an apartment without a microwave.
- Inadequate energy intake related to fear of vomiting and limited variety as evidenced by patient report of five accepted foods that make up regular diet (Pop Tarts, chicken tenders, plain toast, bananas, green beans), daily intake of less than 1,500 calories per day per 24-hour recall, and significant distress (eight out of 10 with 10 being highest) when asked to consume foods outside of accepted items.
- Inadequate energy intake related to increased energy needs of nutritional rehabilitation and fear of weight gain, as evidenced by statement "There's no way I'm eating more than 1,200 calories a day."
- Inadequate oral intake related to economic constraints that limit food availability and storage capacity, as evidenced by recent job loss and patient report of the electricity being turned off in the home.

- Inadequate oral intake related to off-label use of semaglutide, as evidenced by daily energy intake less than 500 kcal.
- Inadequate oral intake related to diagnosis of multiple sclerosis and difficulty preparing food without assistance, as evidenced by patient report of eating only once per day and reported daily intake less than 40% of estimated energy needs.
- Inadequate carbohydrate intake related to adhering to "keto" dietary pattern as evidenced by patient's attempt to exclude all grains, grain products, fruits, and dairy products.
- Inadequate fluid intake related to participation in a weight-class sport as evidenced by stated fear of weight gain, refusal to drink any beverage, report of dizziness upon standing, and dark yellow urine.
- Inadequate dietary fat intake related to harmful beliefs about the effects of fat on the body, as evidenced by avoidance of all foods containing fat and dermatitis consistent with essential fatty acid deficiency.
- Inadequate protein intake related to following a doctor-prescribed vegan diet for weight loss, as evidenced by protein intake at 25% of estimated needs and edema in the lower legs.
- Growth rate below expected related to inconsistent nutrition, as evidenced by no change in height over 1 year and corresponding decrease on growth chart from 75th percentile to 60th percentile.
- Limited access to food related to financial constraints that limit food availability, as evidenced by limited food and beverage intake inconsistent with nutrition reference standards for variety.
- Disordered eating pattern related to diagnosis of attention-deficit with hyperactivity disorder (ADHD), executive dysfunction, and inconsistent response to hunger cues, as evidenced by patient statement "Even if I feel hungry, I get distracted and forget to eat."
- Disordered eating pattern related to harmful beliefs about food as evidenced by avoidance of any food without a nutrition label and using physical activity as a compensatory measure after eating.

- Disordered eating pattern related to caregiver adherence to weight-loss diet as evidenced by limited supply of foods in the home and fear of purchasing additional items for patient's use.
- Disordered eating pattern related to previous experiences in foster care where food was limited and fear of not passing physical testing for military standards due to weight, as evidenced by patient self-report of avoiding all foods containing carbohydrates, secretly stockpiling restricted foods, and binge-eating followed by self-induced vomiting.
- Disordered eating pattern related to restrict-binge-purge cycles (reported four to six times per week) and fear of weight gain, as evidenced by preoccupation with weight (weighing self and body checking up to 60 times per day), and low serum potassium.
- Disordered eating pattern related to gender dysphoria and fears of eating adequately as evidenced by patient statement "They won't do my top surgery until I lose weight," daily reported intake at 60% estimated needs for the past month (1,500 of 2,500 kcal/d per 24-hour recall), and fatigue.
- Disordered eating pattern of daytime restriction and night eating related to shift work, as evidenced by 100% of food intake (approximately 4,000 kcal) consumed within 1 to 2 hours during the night.
- Disordered eating pattern related to desire for weight loss as evidenced by restriction of intake leading to binge eating and intake reflecting an imbalance of macronutrients.
- Excessive physical activity relative to dietary intake related to diagnosis of obsessive-compulsive disorder and body dysmorphia, as evidenced by patient statement "I can see my body getting bigger when I eat," excessive intake of vitamin and mineral supplements, compensatory exercise after meals interfering with work and social life, 6 months since last menstrual cycle, and multiple stress fractures.
- Excessive fluid intake related to diagnosis of anorexia nervosa as evidenced by noncaloric beverage intake at 300% of estimated daily needs and hyponatremia.

- Excessive energy intake related to binge eating while asleep as evidenced by patient report of finding empty food packages upon waking in the morning with no memory of waking or eating.
- Poor nutrition quality of life related to disordered eating pattern as evidenced by compulsion to exercise that interferes with work and social life, fear of eating certain foods, avoidance of social situations that involve food, and excessive amounts of time and energy spent planning meals and exercise.

References

1. Academy of Nutrition and Dietetics. NCP Step 2: Nutrition Diagnosis. eNCPT website. 2023. Accessed January 26, 2024. www.ncpro.org/pubs/2023-encpt-en/category-2

CHAPTER 5

Nutrition Intervention for Eating Disorders: Food and Nutrient Delivery

Nutritional Rehabilitation

The eventual goal of nutrition intervention is nutritional rehabilitation—a restoration (or in some cases, improvement) of preillness nutrition status.[1] This long-range goal will require many short-term nutrition interventions in coordination with medical, social, and emotional needs, situations, and factors. Goals and efforts will be reassessed and revised throughout, and progress may not be easy or linear.

Although nutritional rehabilitation may be elusive, one certainty is that it is not defined solely, or even primarily, by a person's body weight. For most of history, the only recognized eating disorder was anorexia nervosa, and treatment was synonymous with enforced weight gain. Once bulimia and binge-eating disorder were recognized, treatment shifted to "weight normalization," ie, gain or loss toward an "ideal." But eating disorders are not primarily weight disorders, so weight-focused treatment does not solve them. On the contrary, a focus on weight can create new problems without solving the original ones.

Appropriate nutritional rehabilitation is weight-inclusive in two senses: it recognizes that all eating disorders cause malnutrition, regardless of body size; and it incorporates body weight as only one piece of information among many others. This weight-inclusive stance allows a focus on normalization of nutrition parameters and the behaviors that will maintain them, with acknowledgment that weight changes may *accompany* treatment, but are not its only goal, nor evidence that it has succeeded or failed.

Nevertheless, eating disorder specialty programs usually have expectations for the pace of weight gain for emaciated patients. In higher levels of care, such as a hospital or treatment center, more-rapid weight gain is expected, and monitoring is more frequent. Many factors may influence the rate of weight gain in the inpatient setting, including risk of refeeding syndrome (discussed later in this chapter), patient willingness to accept nutrition support, and hypermetabolism, which requires much higher energy intake than standard equations predict. In outpatient care, weight gain may be slower and less consistent.

Nutrition interventions begin with a planning phase that includes prioritization of nutrition intervention(s), collaboration with patients and others to set goals, writing the nutrition prescription, and selecting appropriate intervention strategies. Nutrition interventions may begin with a standard protocol and can then be modified as needed to meet each patient's needs and progress. Modify food and nutrient delivery on an individual basis by monitoring the patient's overall progress, including weight changes, fluid shifts, and medical parameters, and in consultation with other providers.[2]

Food and Nutrient Delivery

Faced with multiple nutrition-related deficiencies and needed interventions, how does a registered dietitian nutritionist (RDN) prioritize? Barring any medical or mental health crisis requiring emergency care, the RDN starts with food and nutrient delivery. Adequate nutrition is required for an individual with an eating disorder to repair the physical and mental damage of malnutrition, implement health-promoting eating practices, and move toward a safe relationship with food and eating.[3] Ensuring that each patient has access to adequate nutrition is a key component of eating disorder treatment in addition to being a social justice issue.

Eating disorders disrupt an individual's internal environment to the point that self-nourishment becomes overwhelming and sometimes impossible. Co-occurring medical and psychiatric conditions, along with the social and environmental aspects that contribute to and reinforce dysfunctional eating behaviors, combine with eating disorder thought processes to impair an individual's ability to follow recommendations even when they intend to.[3-6] RDNs are well aware that planning and providing consistent, balanced, adequate, nutritious, enjoyable, varied, and visually appealing meals that accommodate personal preferences, cultural practices, resources, and abilities is hard enough for an individual who is well. In eating disorder care, maintaining adequate nutrition independently may be a very long-term goal.

The RDN's role in food and nutrient delivery varies widely through the levels of eating disorder care.[4] Higher-intensity treatment (residential, inpatient, and partial hospitalization), where patients have staff support at multiple eating opportunities per day, provides more opportunities for support and guidance than outpatient care and programs. For this reason, an individual's own ability—including availability of in-home support—to meet their own nutrition needs is one of the determining factors in the American Psychiatric Association's (APA) guidelines for determining which level of eating disorder care is appropriate at a given time.[3] Refer to Chapter 8 for levels of care guidelines.

In the more-intensive or high-contact levels of care, the RDN may have full responsibility for diet orders, menus, food preparation, and nutritional quality, while the patient's only responsibility with respect to nutrition is to eat (or not). In less-intensive or lower-contact levels of care, the RDN and patient work together on planning, culinary skills, and implementation. The RDN supplies nutrition knowledge and recommendations about food, and the patient (with the help of support partners, if available) bears more of the responsibility for obtaining, preparing, storing, and consuming it. As a patient transitions through their recovery process, the balance of responsibility may shift back and forth. Experiential opportunities, such as eating together, meal coaching, grocery shopping, and cooking lessons, are optional interventions that may assist an individual in moving toward independent food and nutrient delivery.

Box 5.1 lists general guidelines that can be used as initial recommendations for food and nutrient delivery in any level of care. As with all aspects of medical nutrition therapy, ongoing recommendations should be made on an individual basis by the RDN.

BOX 5.1 Food and Nutrient Delivery Guidelines for Eating Disorders: Meals and Snacks

Food and nutrient delivery parameter	*Guidelines specific to all eating disorders*
Eating opportunities	Three or more per day, depending on nutrition needs and volume tolerated each time.
Meal or snack timing and spacing	Times should be determined in advance and maintained as much as possible day to day. Take into account patient's work or school schedule (LL).[a] Avoid lengthy periods >3 hours (HL) or >4 hours (LL) between eating opportunities to prevent drops in blood glucose or excessive hunger, except during sleep. Consider bedside snack if waking to eat.
Meal or snack size and volume	Use current intake as a base. If inadequate, increase by 100 to 200 calories daily (HL) or 200 to 500 calories weekly (LL). To reduce volume, discourage noncaloric and carbonated beverages, high-fiber, nutrient poor, or low-calorie "filler" foods, and offer small portions of nutrient-dense foods to avoid gastrointestinal distress and impulse to purge. Use nutrition supplements as needed between eating opportunities until higher volume is tolerated.

Continued on next page

Food and Nutrient Delivery

BOX 5.1 Food and Nutrient Delivery Guidelines for Eating Disorders: Meals and Snacks (cont.)

Food and nutrient delivery parameter	*Guidelines specific to all eating disorders*
Meal or snack content	Include protein, carbohydrate, and fat sources at each meal. Exclude confirmed allergens, religion-prohibited foods, and medically prohibited foods such as gluten, if applicable. As much as possible, use preferred foods in amounts that meet macronutrient needs. If additional foods must be added to meet needs, use least-challenging foods to lessen anxiety. Advance toward balance and variety going from least to most challenging foods as tolerated. Exclude foods known to cause reflux or gastrointestinal distress if possible. Exclude foods historically binged or purged, and foods associated with emotional distress or self-harming behaviors unless supervision is available.
Beverages	Avoid carbonated beverages if they are used to induce vomiting. Assess report of excessive thirst as possible medication side-effect. Discourage or limit caffeinated beverage intake due to appetite suppressive effect. Consider weaning schedule for caffeine dependence.
Meal or snack duration	Consider a guideline for appropriate meal duration to promote appropriate pace of eating; extend or decrease eating time as needed.

BOX 5.1 Food and Nutrient Delivery Guidelines for Eating Disorders: Meals and Snacks (cont.)

Food and nutrient delivery parameter	*Guidelines specific to all eating disorders*
Meal or snack supervision and support	Consider supervision or support while eating to discourage hiding, concealing, or chewing and spitting food. Consider supervision or support after eating to discourage purging or other self-harming behaviors. Consider support after eating to process feelings of distress. If meal preparation or cleanup trigger binge eating, delegate these tasks to others or provide supervision or support.
Meal or snack behavior	Discourage food rituals and conversation about food and food content. Implement mindful eating or stress-management practices as appropriate before, during, or after eating. Consider gentle guidance during meals to speed up or slow pace of eating, avoid ritualistic eating behaviors, and encourage social interaction. If gentle guidance triggers shame, consider providing it during a meal processing or nutrition counseling session instead.
Meal or snack documentation	Document food and beverage intake, compensatory behaviors, and any other information to assist in continued treatment planning.

[a] Indicates when a recommendation is specific to higher levels (HL) vs lower levels (LL) of care.

Oral Nutrition Supplements

Oral nutrition supplements (ONS), such as fortified beverages and puddings, can be used for food and nutrient delivery in eating disorder care. Some specific benefits of ONS include:

- They increase energy and macronutrient intake beyond what an individual is willing or able to ingest from food. This is especially true for high-calorie (>1 kcal/mL) ONS options.
- They are consistent in taste and texture (although they may not be palatable for someone sensitive to taste or smell).
- They do not require biting or chewing. This may be helpful for someone who has pain or sores in the mouth (associated with vomiting), tooth loss (associated with malnutrition), or texture aversions (associated with avoidant/restrictive food intake disorder).
- They supply a balance of micronutrients to compensate for limited food variety.
- They provide a concrete reminder that eating is a necessity, not a luxury, to someone who is averse to eating foods they enjoy. (A fear of enjoying food can be a symptom of any eating disorder and may stem from a fear of overeating, feeling "out of control" or gluttonous, social conditioning that tasty food is unhealthy, or other reasons.)
- They offer relief from some of the decision-making fatigue associated with eating disorder recovery.

As with all aspects of medical nutrition therapy for eating disorders, ONS should be provided as a supportive intervention, never an aversive or punitive one. The RDN should specify if ONS should be used as a meal replacement or in addition to a meal; and at what point before, during, after, or between meals they should be provided.

Use of ONS is highly individual and without standard protocols. What is the appropriate length of time to offer ONS? When should they be discontinued? When a patient is meeting 75% of nutrition needs with food? 90%? Should an RDN insist that a patient rely on food rather than allowing ONS use? No standard of care or best practice for use of ONS exists. As with many aspects of eating disorder care, a decision should be made on a case-by-case basis and together with each patient, their support partners, and other providers.

Some patients will benefit from encouragement to transition from ONS intake to solid food when the time is right; others will wean themselves naturally as their recovery progresses. Some may continue to incorporate ONS into their ongoing eating pattern simply because they like them or find them convenient.

> ***Expert Insight***
>
> *If a patient appears to rely on ONS for nutrition beyond the point that they seem necessary, open a conversation about it. If the patient expresses fear of enjoying food, lack of interest in food due to depression, fear of the caloric uncertainty of solid food, or fear of recovery, consult with the patient's mental health professional or your supervisor for guidance.*

Nutrition Support

Enteral Nutrition

Enteral nutrition (EN) support, including feeding via nasogastric, nasojejunal, nasoduodenal, gastrostomy, or jejunostomy tubes, may be useful any time an individual is unable to adequately eat by mouth. They may be used in three types of scenarios: the eating disorder physically impairs eating or digestion; the eating disorder mentally impairs eating or digestion; or the impairment is unrelated to the eating disorder.

Examples of physical impairment include scenarios when an individual may be experiencing gastroparesis (food does not move out of the stomach in a timely manner, causing nausea, unintentional vomiting, or inability to tolerate the next meal), uncontrollable vomiting (due to damage to the cardiac sphincter, caused by chronic vomiting), or superior mesenteric artery syndrome (the loss of intra-abdominal fat pads resulting in intense pain upon eating).

EN support can also be useful in situations where an individual's digestive tract is intact and functioning, but the mental process of the eating disorder (or other psychiatric condition) prevents them from eating adequately by mouth. EN support may be used as a person's exclusive source of nutrition or on a supplementary basis, as determined by the RDN and depending on the amount and content of the individual's oral intake.

In eating disorder care the determining factor for EN support is not that a patient *could* eat but whether or not they *do* eat.

Very occasionally, the knowledge that tube placement is imminent will motivate a patient to eat more by mouth. This should not be expected, mistaken for recovery, or used as a threat or coercion. As with all aspects of medical nutrition therapy, EN support should be initiated when nutritionally necessary and appropriate, never as a punishment.

As nutritional rehabilitation progresses, ideally psychological and gastrointestinal functioning will improve, the patient's hunger cues restore and are responded to, and oral nutrition intake increases. If this happens, nutrition support can be decreased and ultimately discontinued. However, the real world is far from ideal. Use caution in blaming all digestive distress on an eating disorder or suggesting that the solution is simply nutrition. While there are many examples of digestive problems caused or exacerbated by eating disorders, there are just as many that predate or will outlast it. In cases of permanent damage or chronic and enduring inability to meet nutritional needs by mouth, a gastrostomy or jejunostomy may be needed for long-term nutrition support.

Parenteral Nutrition

In eating disorder treatment, use of parenteral nutrition (PN) is often avoided because it interferes with the ability to sense hunger cues and does not promote the eating behaviors usually required for eating disorder recovery. However PN should be used when necessary, for example when an individual has disconnected, contaminated, refused, or purged their enteral feedings even when supervised, or when they are experiencing bowel obstruction or other digestive issues that prevent oral or enteral feeding.

Box 5.2 provides example scenarios when enteral and parenteral feedings might be used in eating disorder care.[3,6,7]

BOX 5.2 Nutrition Support in Eating Disorders: Case Studies[3,6,7]

Patient case #1

After Dakari was told by his school nurse that he needed to lose weight, he burned his tongue on purpose so that he wouldn't be tempted to eat. He was admitted to the hospital through the emergency room after friends told his parents he had not eaten for 3 days.

Each time foodservice brings Dakari a tray, he says he's not hungry and won't allow it to be brought into the room. He was offered liquid nutritional supplements but will not drink them. Twenty-four hours after admission, Dakari's only recorded oral intake is a few sips of water.

Sample recommendation

Initiate continuous drip tube feeding of isocaloric formula at a rate of 30 mL/h. If tolerated × 8 hours, switch to intermittent feedings over 20 minutes every mealtime, starting with 120 mL and advancing in 60 mL increments as tolerated until reaching goal rate of 240 mL per feed. Run continuous overnight feed of 30 mL per hour from 10 PM to 6 AM.

Continue to offer meal trays and the option of substituting an oral supplement at breakfast, lunch, afternoon snack, and dinner times. Hold tube feeding (TF) at any mealtime patient eats >50% of tray or drinks >50% of oral supplement. Discontinue TF when patient is able to eat >75% of every meal × 3 days.

Continued on next page

BOX 5.2 Nutrition Support in Eating Disorders: Case Studies[3,6,7] (cont.)

Patient case #2

Yaretzi was diagnosed with bulimia nervosa (BN) 2 months ago and has been working with an outpatient team. She has been mostly successful in overcoming her urges to induce vomiting but has not been eating enough because even a small amount of food intake leads to intense nausea.

Yaretzi was admitted to the hospital for observation after fainting at work. Very motivated to be discharged, she rapidly ate a large meal and almost immediately vomited.

Testing has revealed that she is experiencing gastroparesis.

Sample recommendation

Trial a slow (30 mL/hour) 24-hour continuous nasojejunal tube (NJ) feeding of an isocaloric formula and advance as tolerated to maintenance calories, switching to a 1.5 kcal/mL formula if needed.

Continue to provide six trays per day with small portions of bland, low-fat, low-fiber foods. No low-calorie foods or beverages. Encourage patient to eat slowly and only if tolerated.

Once patient is able to eat small amounts during the day, discontinue TF from breakfast through dinner. Continue to run TF at night until patient is able to meet nutrition needs by mouth (PO).

Patient case #3

Theo was admitted to an eating disorder residential program due to his fear of eating, reluctance to stop exercising, and inability to gain weight as recommended by his cardiologist.

Because he is no longer able to purge via compensatory exercise, he is only able to eat small amounts at meals. His weight continues to drop, and he now reports feeling dizzy when standing as well as chest palpitations.

Sample recommendation

Initiate overnight nasogastric tube (NG) tube feeding per refeeding protocol and advance as tolerated to 120 mL per hour continuous with a 1.5 kcal/mL formula starting at hour of sleep (HS) until 4 hours before breakfast.

Offer regular meals and snacks with a nutrition supplement as a beverage. Staff to document all food and beverage intake. Dietitian will monitor intake, weight, and vital signs to determine whether to increase nighttime TF rate.

BOX 5.2 Nutrition Support in Eating Disorders: Case Studies[3,6,7] (cont.)

Patient case #4

Eloisa was brought to the emergency department by her roommate who was alarmed when Eloisa didn't eat, sleep, or go to work for 3 days in a row. A computed tomography (CT) scan and toxicology screen, ordered because Eloisa had slurred speech and was unable to answer the triage nurse's questions coherently, were both negative, so a psychiatry consult was ordered. After reviewing the medical record, the psychiatry fellow pointed out that Eloisa's labs and vital signs suggested severe malnutrition, even though, as the triage nurse said, "It's not like she's underweight." Eloisa remained in the emergency department while the triage nurse tried to discharge her and Eloisa's roommate refused to take her home. Eventually she was admitted to the general psychiatry unit.

Sample recommendation

Initiate NG tube feeding per standard facility protocol and advance as tolerated to provide total energy needs over a 24-hour period via continuous drip.

Once 100% of daily nutrient needs are being met via TF, divide by 6 and advance as tolerated to bolus feedings at meal and snack times to promote a normal pattern of hunger.

Offer preferred foods and nutrition supplement beverage in response to any expressions of desire by patient to eat or drink PO. Decrease TF as voluntary intake improves. Discontinue TF when patient is meeting nutrition needs PO.

Patient case #5

Kofi is on the track team and believes that the leaner you are, the faster you can run. Ever since he was teased for being chubby as a kid, he's viewed himself as being "too big," so he didn't realize how much weight he had lost this year until his track coach pointed out he could see his hip bones and pulled Kofi from the team. He was admitted to an eating disorder partial hospitalization program which he attends during the day and then sleeps at home. He is very motivated to eat whatever he needs to in order to go to college in the fall, so he is eating everything on his meal plan and drinking supplements, but it's impossible for him to eat enough to restore weight.

Continued on next page

BOX 5.2 Nutrition Support in Eating Disorders: Case Studies[3,6,7] (cont.)

Sample recommendation

Initiate nighttime home NG tube feeding of 2 kcal/mL formula per refeeding protocol and increase as tolerated to provide 2,500 kcal over 8 hours.

Nurse educator to teach parents how to hook up, run, detach, and flush pump and tube.

Allow the patient to eat ad lib and drink preferred protein shakes throughout the day. Discontinue tube feeding when metabolic rate normalizes and the patient is able to meet 100% of energy needs PO.

Patient case #6

Nhean is an adult autistic male recently diagnosed with binge-eating disorder (BED). He lives in a group home where he is learning to manage his eating disorder with the help of supportive staff. The house manager called 911 when Nhean collapsed in pain one evening. He was admitted to the hospital with a diagnosis of bowel obstruction.

Sample recommendation

Make patient nothing by mouth (NPO) and initiate parenteral nutrition (PN) to meet 100% of nutrient needs until medical team determines that bowel obstruction has resolved.

Patient case #7

Namine attends a therapeutic boarding school for teens. They have a history of multiple adverse experiences in foster care and as a ward of the state. In different hospitals and treatment facilities since the age of 4, Namine has received diagnoses of avoidant/restrictive food intake disorder (ARFID), obsessive-compulsive disorder (OCD), and oppositional defiant disorder (ODD), among others. Currently they have been admitted to a locked psychiatric facility after a violent attack on another student. During the altercation, Namine's jaw was broken, so they are unable to eat solid food. They removed their own NG tube due to expressed discomfort and state they will do the same if it is replaced.

Sample recommendation

Initiate PN to meet 100% of nutrient needs. Allow patient to drink oral nutrition supplement through a straw if desired and if it does not cause discomfort to their injured area. Discuss with social worker whether Namine can return to boarding school with PN or if other arrangements will need to be made for the duration of their recuperation period.

Refeeding Syndrome

Any individual who has become malnourished through starvation or restrictive eating can experience gastrointestinal distress and other symptoms as their body adjusts to nutritional rehabilitation.[7-13] Some symptoms are uncomfortable, such as flatulence, constipation, and nausea, while others are life-threatening. It is these life-threatening symptoms, such as electrolyte imbalance and heart failure, that are known as *refeeding syndrome*.

Refeeding syndrome can occur when a person who is severely malnourished begins nutritional rehabilitation. In the starved state, electrolyte stores are depleted but serum electrolyte laboratory values may appear normal due to homeostatic adaptations over time. Once the refeeding process begins and nutrients are absorbed, adaptations to starvation are rapidly reversed, revealing the severely depleted electrolyte stores.

Refeeding syndrome is preventable when patients at risk are identified early, electrolyte laboratory values are checked every 1 to 2 days, and oral or intravenous replenishment of phosphorous, potassium, magnesium, calcium, and sodium is provided in accordance with the change in laboratory values.[9-14] This close monitoring is needed only for the first 2 weeks of eating disorder treatment, after which the risk of refeeding syndrome is generally considered to have passed.

The National Institute for Health and Clinical Excellence provides these guidelines for identifying patients most at risk of refeeding syndrome[15]:

Patient has one or more of the following:

- BMI less than 16
- Greater than 15% weight loss in the past 3- to 6-month period
- Little or no nutritional intake for more than 1 day
- Low potassium, phosphate, or magnesium prior to initiating refeeding

Or patient has two or more of the following:

- BMI less than 18.5
- Greater than 10% weight loss in the past 3- to 6-month period

- Little or no nutritional intake for more than 5 days
- A history of alcohol or drug abuse including insulin, chemotherapy, antacids, or diuretics

Although these guidelines reference BMI, refeeding syndrome is more closely correlated with duration and severity of malnutrition than with body weight. Therefore individuals with eating disorders, malabsorption syndromes, celiac disease, and who have had bariatric surgery are at risk of refeeding syndrome regardless of amount of weight lost or current body size.

The American Society for Parenteral and Enteral Nutrition (ASPEN) also provides guidelines for identifying adult and pediatric patients most at risk of refeeding syndrome, as well as parameters to monitor to avoid and, when needed, treat at-risk adults and children.[16] The consensus recommendations for adults are listed in Box 5.3.

BOX 5.3 ASPEN Consensus Recommendations for Avoidance and Treatment of Refeeding Syndrome in At-Risk Adults

Aspect of care	*Recommendations*
Initiation of calories	Initiate with 100 to 150 g of dextrose or 10 to 20 kcal/kg for the first 24 hours; advance by 33% of goal every 1 to 2 days. This includes enteral as well as parenteral glucose. In patients with moderate to high risk of refeeding syndrome with low electrolyte levels, holding the initiation or increase of calories until electrolytes are supplemented and/or normalized should be considered. Initiation of or increasing calories should be delayed in patients with severely low phosphorus, potassium, or magnesium levels until corrected.

BOX 5.3 ASPEN Consensus Recommendations for Avoidance and Treatment of Refeeding Syndrome in At-Risk Adults (cont.)

Initiation of calories (cont.)	Calories from intravenous (IV) dextrose solutions and medications being infused in dextrose should be considered in the limits above and/or initiated with caution in patients at moderate to severe risk for refeeding syndrome. If a patient has received significant amounts of dextrose for several days, from maintenance IV fluids and/or medications in dextrose, and has been asymptomatic with stable electrolytes, calories from nutrition may be reintroduced at a higher amount than recommended above.
Fluid restriction	No recommendation.
Sodium restriction	No recommendation.
Protein restriction	No recommendation.
Electrolytes	Check serum potassium, magnesium, and phosphorus before initiation of nutrition. Monitor every 12 hours for the first 3 days in high-risk patients. May be more frequent based on clinical picture. Replete low electrolytes based on established standards of care. No recommendation can be made for whether prophylactic dosing of electrolytes should be given if prefeeding levels are normal. If electrolytes become difficult to correct or drop precipitously during the initiation of nutrition, decrease calories/grams of dextrose by 50% and advance the dextrose/calories by approximately 33% of goal every 1 to 2 days based on clinical presentation. Recommendations may be changed based on practitioner judgment and clinical presentation, and cessation of nutrition support may be considered when electrolyte levels are severely and/or life-threateningly low or dropping precipitously.

Continued on next page

BOX 5.3 ASPEN Consensus Recommendations for Avoidance and Treatment of Refeeding Syndrome in At-Risk Adults (cont.)

Thiamin and multivitamins	Supplement thiamin 100 mg before feeding or before initiating dextrose-containing IV fluids in patients at risk. Supplement thiamin 100 mg/d for 5 to 7 days or longer in patients with severe starvation, chronic alcoholism, or other high risk for deficiency and/or signs of thiamin deficiency. Multivitamin is added to parenteral nutrition (PN) daily, unless contraindicated, as long as PN is continued. For patients receiving oral/enteral nourishment, add complete oral/enteral multivitamin once daily for 10 days or greater based on clinical status and mode of therapy.
Monitoring and long-term care	Recommend vital signs every 4 hours for the first 24 hours after initiation of calories in patients at risk. Cardiorespiratory monitoring is recommended for unstable patients or those with severe deficiencies, based on established standards of care. Daily weights with monitored intake and output. Evaluate short- and long-term goals for nutrition care daily during the first several days until the patient is deemed stabilized (eg, no requirement for electrolyte supplementation for 2 days) and then based on institutional standards of care.

Adapted with permission from reference 16: da Silva JSV, Seres DS, Sabino K, et al. ASPEN consensus recommendations for refeeding syndrome. *Nutr Clin Pract*. 2020;35(2):178-195. doi:10.1002/ncp.10474

Vitamin and Mineral Supplementation

There are infinite varieties of liked, disliked, avoided, and accepted foods, and no two individuals will have the same list. There is no way to generalize or predict micronutrient deficiencies based on diagnosis or patient profile, and laboratory values are often within normal limits until deficiencies become severe. There are no standard protocols for micronutrient supplementation, although many eating disorder care facilities provide a multivitamin/mineral supplement to all patients. The best way to determine which micronutrients an individual might lack is to evaluate which foods are being avoided.

Box 5.4 summarizes the micronutrients that may be deficient in patients who have eliminated most or all foods in a certain food group.

Table 5.1 on page 110 summarizes the available data on single-nutrient supplementation for individuals with eating disorders.[16,17]

BOX 5.4 Potential Micronutrient Deficiencies Caused by Food Group Restriction

Restricted or eliminated food group	*Micronutrients potentially deficient*
Dairy products	Calcium, vitamin D, vitamin B12
Vegetables	Fiber, potassium, folic acid, vitamin C
Meat, poultry, fish, eggs	Iron, zinc, selenium, magnesium, copper, vitamin B12, omega-3 fatty acids
Fats, oils	Vitamins E, A, and D; omega-3 fatty acids
Grains (bread, cereal, rice, pasta)	B vitamins
Fruits	Vitamins A and C, folic acid, potassium

TABLE 5.1 Micronutrient Deficiencies and Supplementation Guidelines for Eating Disorders[16,17]

Nutrient	Preferred method to assess deficiency in patients with eating disorders	Eating disorder-specific supplementation guidelines
Calcium[a]	Long-term: poor bone density Short-term: dietary inadequacy	Supplement with calcium citrate to total 1,500 mg/d elemental calcium from food and supplement. Divide calcium dose into 500 mg increments
Iron	Plasma ferritin <30 ng/mL for males and <15 ng/mL for females	Refer to physician for prescription. Long-term administration and monitoring necessary
Phosphate[a]	<2.5 mg/dL	IV administration per patient needs
Potassium[a]	<3.5 mEq/L	IV administration per patient needs
Magnesium[a]	<1.5 mEq/L	IV administration per patient needs
Sodium[a]	<136 mEq/L	IV administration per patient needs
Vitamin A (retinol, carotene)	Dietary inadequacy	700 mcg retinol/d (RDA for females >14 years old) 900 mcg retinol/d (RDA for males >14 years old) Supplementation above the RDA not recommended
Vitamin B1 (thiamin)	Dietary inadequacy Alcohol dependence	100 mg/d for 5-7 d

TABLE 5.1 Micronutrient Deficiencies and Supplementation Guidelines for Eating Disorders[16,17] (cont.)

Nutrient	Preferred method to assess deficiency in patients with eating disorders	Eating disorder-specific supplementation guidelines
Vitamin B2 (riboflavin)	Long-term: activity coefficient of erythrocyte glutathione reductase >1.4 Short-term: dietary inadequacy	1.3 mg/d (RDA for males) 1.1 mg/d (RDA for females)
Vitamin B6 (pyridoxine)	Dietary inadequacy Alcohol dependence	1.3 mg/d
Vitamin B9 (folic acid)	Plasma folate ≤3 ng/mL or red blood cell folate ≤140 ng/mL or elevated plasma homocysteine level	400 mcg/d
Vitamin B12 (cobalamin)	<200 pg/mL or elevated plasma homocysteine level	1 mg intramuscular cyanocobalamin per month or 2 mg oral cyanocobalamin per day
Vitamin C	Long-term: 2-h urinary excretion <28 mg, 4 h after preload of ascorbic acid Short-term: dietary inadequacy	Up to 400 mg/d
Vitamin D	25-hydroxyvitamin D <20 ng/mL	As needed to correct deficiency
Zinc	Serum zinc <46 ng/dL Hypogeusia (diminished sense of taste)	100 mg/d zinc gluconate (providing 14 mg/d elemental zinc)

Abbreviations: IV, intravenous; RDA, Recommended Dietary Allowance

[a]Abnormal blood value levels of these nutrients reflect long-term or serious whole-body deficiency. These should be referred for medical evaluation and should be checked daily during the first week of nutritional rehabilitation as levels can decrease even with supplementation.

Food and Nutrient Delivery

Nutrition-Related Medication Management

Only two medications have been approved to directly treat eating disorders. Fluoxetine has been Food and Drug Administration (FDA) approved to treat bulimia, and lisdexamfetamine has been FDA approved to treat moderate to severe binge-eating disorder.[18] Topiramate and semaglutide have each been trialed as treatments for binge-eating disorder.[19-21] To date, no medications have been approved specifically to treat anorexia nervosa.

Nevertheless, medications are often utilized in eating disorder care. Although not prescribed to counter a specific eating disorder behavior, medications can provide significant support to eating disorder treatment, management, and recovery. When prescribed, dosed, and monitored by a skilled professional, medications that diminish obsessive thoughts and ruminations, decrease paralyzing depression or anxiety, or allow for clearer thinking or concentration, can be an important piece of the mental health puzzle.

Over time, eating disorder symptoms can markedly improve, and in a minority of cases, completely remit. An eating disorder care team cannot be considered complete without a psychiatric practitioner who ideally works with each patient to find the best medication option(s) by monitoring dosages, benefits, and side effects. If the decision is made to decrease or discontinue a medication, all treatment team members including the patient should be alert for any flare-ups in symptoms or behaviors that may occur.

Nutrition-Related Side Effects and Medication Abuse

The RDN's role expands when a psychoactive medication is prescribed. Medication and nutrition influence each other, and medication efficacy may be enhanced or reduced depending on nutrition status. Not every person will experience every medication side effect; nevertheless, it is helpful for the RDN to be aware of potential concerns and to counsel the individual accordingly. Encourage patients to report all side effects (nutrition-related and otherwise) to the prescribing provider.

The RDN may have the most-frequent contact with the patient, particularly in the outpatient setting, and may recognize medication side effects that patients are attributing to increased eating or to certain foods. Appropriately ascribing these side effects (such as gastrointestinal distress) to medications rather than food can improve the patient's willingness to continue nutritional rehabilitation.

Many medications affect appetite and thirst, yet patients are not always educated about these side effects by their prescriber. The RDN plays an important role in helping patients manage these side effects. For example, they may recommend increased water intake rather than high-calorie beverages to manage dry mouth. Medications that decrease appetite, such as stimulants, provide the greatest challenge for individuals who need to increase their nutritional intake. Confer with the prescribing professional to determine if the medication timing can be moved from before eating to after eating or made entirely separate from mealtime.

Patients who induce vomiting immediately or a short time after taking their medication may not receive the full effects of their medication. This should be addressed either via changing the timing of meals, the timing of medication (with supervision of the prescribing professional), or behavioral intervention.

Medications that impact weight, whether as an intended or unintended effect, provide specific challenges in our weight-obsessed society. Medication-induced weight change should be reported to the prescribing professional. In some cases, alternatives exist. In others, the benefits of the medication supersede its effects on weight. Patients may need additional encouragement to continue taking a needed medication that causes unwanted weight gain or to discontinue an inappropriate medication that causes dangerous weight loss.

Certain medications are weight-dependent and may require adjustment of dosages with major changes in weight. Regardless of their cause, report large weight changes over time to the prescribing physician.

When a patient reports undesirable side effects or expresses a desire to discontinue a prescribed medication, encourage them to speak with their prescriber rather than abruptly stop taking it. Some substances build up in the bloodstream over time and require a weaning protocol to avoid complications. If a patient reports noncompliance with medication to you (overdosing or underdosing or use other than as prescribed), or that they have run out of a prescribed medication, you or the patient should report this right away to a member of the medical team who can advise the patient.

Some patients with eating disorders abuse prescription or over-the-counter medications. This should be reported to the psychiatrist on the team, or a referral should be made if the patient has not had a psychiatric evaluation. Although inappropriate, this type of drug use may point to a legitimate need for medication. There is one important exception: an individual abusing ipecac syrup as a means to induce vomiting should be counseled to stop immediately, and the physician should be notified. Ipecac syrup builds up in the body and can be lethal.

Box 5.5 includes selected medications and their known potential nutrition-related effects.[3,6,20,22-24]

BOX 5.5 Nutrition-Related Medication Side Effects[3,6,20,22-24]

Medication (brand name)	*FDA[a]-approved for treatment of*	*Potential drug-nutrient interactions and side effects*
Alprazolam (Xanax)	Anxiety	Appetite increase or decrease Weight increase or decrease
Aripiprazole (Abilify)	Bipolar disorder Schizophrenia Depression	Weight increase Nausea Constipation Hyperglycemia Orthostatic hypotension
Amitriptyline (Elavil)	Anxiety Depression	Appetite increase Weight increase Carbohydrate and sweets cravings Increased blood glucose levels High fiber intake may decrease drug efficacy Increased need for riboflavin

Food and Nutrient Delivery

BOX 5.5 Nutrition-Related Medication Side Effects[3,6,20,22-24] (cont.)

Medication (brand name)	*FDA-approved for treatment of*	*Potential drug-nutrient interactions and side effects*
Amphetamine salts (Adderall)[b]	Attention deficit hyperactivity disorder (ADHD)	Appetite decrease (can be dramatic) Weight decrease (can be dramatic) Difficulty gaining weight
Bupropion (Wellbutrin)	Depression Smoking cessation	Appetite decrease Weight decrease
Buspirone (BuSpar)	Anxiety	Nausea Diarrhea
Carbamaze-pine (Tegretol, Equetro)	Bipolar disorder	Appetite decrease
Chlorpromazine (Thorazine)	Schizophrenia Anxiety	Appetite increase Weight increase Increased cholesterol levels Increased blood glucose levels Increased need for riboflavin Cardiac complications
Citalopram (Celexa)	Depression	Weight increase possible
Clonazepam (Klonopin)	Anxiety	Appetite decrease Weight increase or decrease Increased thirst

Continued on next page

BOX 5.5 Nutrition-Related Medication Side Effects[3,6,20,22-24] (cont.)

Medication (brand name)	*FDA-approved for treatment of*	*Potential drug-nutrient interactions and side effects*
Clozapine (Clozaril)	Schizophrenia Anxiety	Weight increase (can be extreme) Severe constipation Cardiac complications Increased blood glucose levels Increased cholesterol levels New-onset diabetes mellitus
Desipramine (Norpramin)	Anxiety Depression	Appetite increase Weight increase Sweets cravings High-fiber diet may decrease drug efficacy Increased need for riboflavin Increased glucose levels
Dextroamphetamine (Dexedrine)[b]	ADHD	Appetite decrease Weight decrease Calcium or magnesium supplements may increase drug effect Vitamin C supplement or acidic foods may decrease drug absorption
Doxepin (Sinequan, Adapin)	Anxiety Depression	Appetite increase Weight increase Increased thirst Sweets cravings High-fiber diet may decrease efficacy Increased blood glucose levels

Food and Nutrient Delivery

BOX 5.5 Nutrition-Related Medication Side Effects[3,6,20,22-24] (cont.)

Medication (brand name)	*FDA-approved for treatment of*	*Potential drug-nutrient interactions and side effects*
Duloxetine (Cymbalta)	Depression	Appetite increase or decrease Weight increase or decrease
Escitalopram (Lexapro)	Depression	Appetite increase Weight increase Increased cholesterol levels
Fluoxetine (Prozac)	Anxiety Depression Bulimia	Appetite increase Weight increase
Flurazepam (Dalmane)	Insomnia	Appetite increase or decrease Weight increase or decrease
Fluvoxamine (Luvox)	Obsessive-compulsive disorder Bulimia Schizophrenia Panic disorder	Appetite increase or decrease Weight increase or decrease Increased cholesterol levels
Lithium (Eskalith, Lithotabs, Lithonate, Lithane)	Bipolar disorder	Weight increase Appetite decrease Increased thirst Increased serum electrolyte levels Bloating Limit xanthine (coffee, tea, cola) Recommend noncaloric beverages and consistent sodium intake
Lisdexamfetamine (Vyvanse)[b]	ADHD Binge eating disorder	Appetite decrease (can be dramatic) Weight decrease (can be dramatic) Nausea

Continued on next page

BOX 5.5 Nutrition-Related Medication Side Effects[3,6,20,22-24] (cont.)

Medication (brand name)	*FDA-approved for treatment of*	*Potential drug-nutrient interactions and side effects*
Lurasidone (Latuda)	Bipolar disorder	Nausea
Methylphenidate (Ritalin)[b]	ADHD	Appetite decrease (can be dramatic) Weight decrease (can be dramatic) Difficulty gaining weight
Nortriptyline (Pamelor)	Anxiety Depression	Appetite increase Weight increase Carbohydrate and sweets cravings Increased blood glucose levels High fiber intake may decrease drug efficacy Increased need for riboflavin
Olanzapine (Zyprexa)	Schizophrenia Anxiety	Appetite increase Weight increase (can be dramatic and can cause diabetes or ketosis) Increased cholesterol or triglyceride levels Cardiac complications
Paroxetine (Paxil)	Anxiety Depression	Appetite increase (can be dramatic) Weight increase (can be dramatic)
Pemoline (Cylert)	ADHD	Appetite decrease (can be dramatic) Weight loss or difficulty gaining weight

BOX 5.5 Nutrition-Related Medication Side Effects[3,6,20,22-24] (cont.)

Medication (brand name)	*FDA-approved for treatment of*	*Potential drug-nutrient interactions and side effects*
Phenelzine (Nardil)	Depression	Appetite increase Weight increase Monoamine oxidase inhibitor (MAOI)—limit high tyramine foods
Phenytoin (Dilantin)	Antiseizure	Decreased folate, phosphorus, cholesterol, calcium, vitamin D levels Increased blood glucose levels Increased metabolism of vitamins D and K Folic acid supplement >5 mg/wk lowers drug availability Antacids, enteral feedings, and calcium supplements should be separated from drug administration by at least 2 h
Quetiapine (Seroquel)	Bipolar disorder Schizophrenia	Weight increase Constipation Increased glucose and cholesterol levels
Risperidone (Risperdal)	Schizophrenia Anxiety	Appetite increase Weight increase Sodium, hemoglobin, hematocrit levels down Cardiac complications Increased glucose levels

Continued on next page

BOX 5.5 Nutrition-Related Medication Side Effects[3,6,20,22-24] (cont.)

Medication (brand name)	***FDA-approved for treatment of***	***Potential drug-nutrient interactions and side effects***
Semaglutide (Ozempic, Rybelsus, Wegovy)[b]	Type 2 diabetes	Appetite decrease (can be extreme) Nausea Vomiting Diarrhea Constipation Delayed gastric emptying (can be extreme) Gastroparesis
Sertraline (Zoloft)	Anxiety Depression	Appetite increase or decrease Weight increase or decrease Gastrointestinal upset
Thioridazine (Mellaril)	Schizophrenia Anxiety	Appetite increase Weight increase Increased cholesterol and glucose levels Increased need for riboflavin Cardiac complications
Thiothixene (Navane)	Schizophrenia Anxiety	Appetite increase Weight increase Increased need for riboflavin Cardiac complications
Tirzepetide (Mounjaro)[b]	Type 2 diabetes	Appetite decrease (can be extreme) Nausea, vomiting Diarrhea Constipation Delayed gastric emptying Gastroparesis Hypoglycemia

BOX 5.5 Nutrition-Related Medication Side Effects[3,6,20,22-24] (cont.)

Medication (brand name)	***FDA-approved for treatment of***	***Potential drug-nutrient interactions and side effects***
Topiramate (Topamax)	Binge-eating disorder	Decreased impulse to binge Appetite decrease Weight decrease Increased lactic acid levels Metabolic acidosis Kidney stones
Trazodone (Desyrel)	Depression Insomnia	Appetite increase or decrease Weight increase or decrease Anemia Edema
Valproic acid (Depakote)	Bipolar disorder	Appetite increase Weight increase Increased cholesterol levels False-positive ketones test results Gastrointestinal distress Polycystic ovary syndrome Altered thyroid function tests
Venlafaxine (Effexor)	Anxiety Depression Panic disorder	Appetite increase or decrease Weight increase or decrease
Zolpidem (Ambien)	Insomnia	Binge eating or night eating with amnesia, leading to weight gain

[a] FDA = US Food and Drug Administration .

[b] Due to their dramatic appetite-suppressant effects, these medications are vulnerable to abuse.

References

1. Moisey LL, Merriweather JL, Drover JW. The role of nutrition rehabilitation in the recovery of survivors of critical illness: underrecognized and underappreciated. *Crit Care*. 2022;26(1):270. doi:10.1186/s13054-022-04143-5
2. Academy of Nutrition and Dietetics. NCP Step 3: Nutrition Intervention. eNCPT website. 2023. Accessed July 31, 2024. www.ncpro.org/pubs/2023-encpt-en/category-3
3. Yager J, et al. *Practice Guideline for the Treatment of Patients With Eating Disorders, Third Edition*. American Psychiatric Association; 2010. Accessed July 1, 2024. www.psychiatryonline.org/pb/assets/raw/sitewide/practice_guidelines/guidelines/eatingdisorders.pdf
4. Hackert AN, Kniskern MA, Beasley TM. Academy of Nutrition and Dietetics: Revised 2020 Standards of Practice and Standards of Professional Performance for Registered Dietitian Nutritionists (Competent, Proficient, and Expert) in Eating Disorders. *J Acad Nutr Diet*. 2020;120(11):1902-1919.e54. doi:10.1016/j.jand.2020.07.014
5. Reiter CS, Graves L. Nutrition therapy for eating disorders. *Nutr Clin Pract*. 2010;25(2):122-136. doi:10.1177/0884533610361606
6. Setnick J. *The Eating Disorders Clinical Pocket Guide*. 2nd Ed. Understanding Nutrition; 2013.
7. Caggiani C. Using enteral feeding to support eating disorder recovery. *SCAN's Pulse*. 1999:12-14.
8. Woods BK, Runyan B, Lamb RP. Perspectives in nasogastric feeding the eating disorder patient. *Childhood Obesity and Nutrition*. 2009;1(5):257-261.
9. Sachs K, Andersen D, Sommer J, Winkelman A, Mehler PS. Avoiding medical complications during the refeeding of patients with anorexia nervosa. *Eat Disord*. 2015;23(5):411-421. doi:10.1080/10640266.2014.1000111
10. Hofer M, Pozzi A, Joray M, et al. Safe refeeding management of anorexia nervosa inpatients: an evidence-based protocol. *Nutrition*. 2014;30(5):524-530. doi:10.1016/j.nut.2013.09.019
11. Rocks T, Pelly F, Wilkinson P. Nutrition therapy during initiation of refeeding in underweight children and adolescent inpatients with anorexia nervosa: a systematic review of the evidence. *J Acad Nutr Diet*. 2014;114(6):897-907. doi:10.1016/j.jand.2013.11.022
12. Agostino H, Erdstein J, Di Meglio G. Shifting paradigms: continuous nasogastric feeding with high caloric intakes in anorexia nervosa. *J Adolesc Health*. 2013;53(5):590-594. doi:10.1016/j.jadohealth.2013.06.005

13. Tresley J, Sheean PM. Refeeding syndrome: recognition is the key to prevention and management. *J Am Diet Assoc*. 2008;108(12):2105-2108. doi:10.1016/j.jada.2008.09.015
14. Koutsavlis A, Forzley EM, Johnson M, Oakley MA, Trees N, Mehler P. Practical methods for refeeding patients with anorexia nervosa. *Integrative Food, Nutrition and Metabolism*. 2017;4(3):1-5. doi:10.15761/IFNM.1000179
15. National Institute for Health and Clinical Excellence. *Guideline for the Management of Refeeding Syndrome (Adults)*. 2nd ed. NHS Foundation Trust; 2009.
16. da Silva JSV, Seres DS, Sabino K, et al. ASPEN consensus recommendations for refeeding syndrome. *Nutr Clin Pract*. 2020;35(2):178-195. doi:10.1002/ncp.10474
17. Setnick J. Micronutrient deficiencies and supplementation in anorexia and bulimia nervosa: a review of literature. *Nutr Clin Pract*. 2010;25(2):137-142. doi:10.1177/0884533610361478
18. Bello NT, Yeomans BL. Safety of pharmacotherapy options for bulimia nervosa and binge eating disorder. *Expert Opin Drug Saf*. 2018;17(1):17-23. doi:10.1080/14740338.2018.1395854
19. Leombruni P, Lavagnino L, Fassino S. Treatment of obese patients with binge eating disorder using topiramate: a review. *Neuropsychiatr Dis Treat*. 2009;5:385-392. doi:10.2147/ndt.s3420
20. McElroy SL, Hudson JI, Capece JA, et al. Topiramate for the treatment of binge eating disorder associated with obesity: a placebo-controlled study. *Biol Psychiatry*. 2007;61(9):1039-1048. doi:10.1016/j.biopsych.2006.08.008
21. Richards J, Bang N, Ratliff EL, et al. Successful treatment of binge eating disorder with the GLP-1 agonist semaglutide: a retrospective cohort study. *Obes Pillars*. 2023;7:100080. doi:10.1016/j.obpill.2023.100080
22. Pronsky ZM, Crowe JP. *Food Medication Interactions*. 16th ed. Food Medication Interactions; 2010.
23. Stein K. When essential medications provoke new health problems: the metabolic effects of second-generation antipsychotics. *J Am Diet Assoc*. 2010;110(7):992-1001. doi:10.1016/j.jada.2010.05.015
24. McCabe-Sellers BJ, Skipper A; American Dietetic Association. Position of the American Dietetic Association: integration of medical nutrition therapy and pharmacotherapy. *J Am Diet Assoc*. 2010;110(6):950-956. doi:10.1016/j.jada.2010.04.017

CHAPTER 6

Nutrition Intervention for Eating Disorders: Nutrition Education

The mental processes of eating disorders—what the Nutrition Care Process refers to as "harmful beliefs about food and eating"—can resemble fixed delusions, meaning they follow their own internal logic that facts and evidence cannot refute. Because of this, nutrition education will be more effective when provided in response to a specific patient's needs and symptoms, and drawing on their own experience, rather than in a generic or preplanned curriculum.

Food rules and harmful behaviors develop in individuals experiencing eating disorders because they are helpful in some way. When a particular behavior or belief has helped someone organize chaotic thoughts or home life, manage their anxiety, survive food insecurity, or keep their job, providing the correct information is not enough to change behavior. It goes without saying that we should never mock or shame an individual for their mistaken beliefs about food, and we should discourage support partners from doing so. Nutrition education can only free a person from their food rules if they have another way to meet their needs.

Nutrition Education Topics

Weight

Of all the nutrition education topics related to eating disorders, body weight is probably the most compelling and complicated. An individual patient's weight can be discussed and dissected from as many angles as there are people involved, to the point that it can become a distraction or even a barrier to recovery.

Every registered dietitian nutritionist (RDN) knows weight changes and trends are more significant than an individual weight, weight does not change at a predictable pace, and the only thing that changes overnight is hydration. But many patients, support partners, insurance representatives, and even other health care providers often do not know these facts. They may view weight as a proxy for health, recovery, failure, proof that they are good enough, that their child will be okay, or for evidence that the patient is finished with treatment. And this is not unique to eating disorders. Our entire culture is obsessed with weight. As a result, it feels like dietitian vs the world to say, "Weight isn't as important as you think. And it's never as important as nutrition."

Nutrition recommendations are ultimately weight-neutral. Eating disorders cause malnutrition, mental distress, and physical harm. Recovery therefore requires consistent nutrition over days, weeks, and probably months. This may result in weight change—in some cases it is essential, in others not ideal. But how fast that will happen, how long it will take, what weight is the best ... these are not answerable questions.

Recent and past weight history can provide helpful information for what *may* be reasonable to expect, but it is not appropriate to assume a preeating disorder weight as a goal. There may have been bone loss and muscle loss, aging and growth, disability, breast reduction, amputation, etc. Even if an individual's former body weight seems "reasonable," that is no guarantee that their nutrition was as well. Guide everyone to look ahead toward a "new normal" rather than longing for how they were in the past. This is easier when focusing on nutrition and eating behavior with weight as an unknown variable, rather than a goal. Weight changes provide information, not verdicts. Slow changes may contribute to health, and sudden shifts may be harmful. Surprising developments deserve investigation. But ultimately, and perhaps disappointingly, weight is an autonomous body function. It cannot be controlled nor relied on as a sole determining factor of health. This is going to be a challenging concept to convey in our weight-obsessed field in our weight-obsessed society.

A related category of nutrition education hinges on the invented concept of "ideal body weight," closely related to BMI. When these topics arise, explain that they are like dinosaurs—extinct. Not only are they passé, their origins are racist, classist, and unscientific. The idea that there is a fixed number at which each person will find "health" is not only faulty but also dangerous. It suggests that this weight is achievable, definable, and something that should be attempted even if it is not safe to do so—in other words, one of the very factors that drives eating disorders.

There is no way to predict the weight at which a given human will be "healthy," considering how many factors play into weight and health that are not within our control. The closest approximation to something like "a healthy weight" would be evidenced by global functioning, influenced by many variables, and changing throughout a lifetime. That is not going to be a predictable number. You would not know until you got there, and then it could change at any time. However, that is not what insurance is after when they ask for a patient's "ideal weight."

For true eating disorder recovery, improved nutrition and nonweight parameters are far more effective and tangible goals. They are individual and measurable, and the benefits are clear; but that does not mean they are easy. They require access to food and safe places to move, financial security, a reasonable workload and adequate childcare, a violence-free home, affordable medicine, dental care and health care, social support, and sometimes in-home nursing or disability care. Suddenly it is clear why focusing on an "ideal weight" is so appealing. It is a total distraction from the actual issues.

As a final reason to avoid discussions of weight, internally ruminating about numbers is part of the mental process of eating disorders. Discussing or debating the numbers fuels the disorder. The best course of action for an RDN is simply to clarify up front that weight is a vital sign that will be monitored but not negotiated, and any deeper attachments to particular numbers should be addressed in a therapeutic setting with a mental health provider.

Even when weight changes are required for recovery, they are unlikely to occur at a predictable or constant rate. This may be disappointing for someone who is highly motivated and frightening for someone who is afraid of change. And this may be the same person! Fear of weight change is often an important topic for nutrition education. Useful aspects to address include:

- Weight is a consequence of many factors occurring over time; one food, one meal, or one day does not have enough power to change it.
- Rapid weight changes are most likely related to hydration status, hormone fluctuations, replenishment of muscle and liver glycogen stores, and the movement of food and fluids through the digestive tract.
- Weight should be expected to change throughout life.
- Weight is an unconscious process, a natural bodily function, that will bend to conscious control only to a point.
- Weight and weight changes are not a reflection of accomplishment or how much someone is working toward recovery. Recovery does not hinge on whether a certain weight goal was met or missed.

When a patient's weight changes or does not change as they hoped it would, they may benefit from reassurance that this is to be expected and does not reflect badly on them. Eating disorder thought processes cause body size and weight to have a disproportionate affect on a person's self-esteem and how they believe others judge them. Weight-inclusive dietitians convey that we value our patients regardless and support any and all beneficial behavior changes whether or not they result in weight change.

Nutrition education about weight can also benefit support partners. It is helpful for individuals who spend time with the patient to hear the same information. Encourage them to view recovery as much more than weight, and that ending treatment when weight seems "back to normal" is not ideal. Regardless of their own stance or choices, a patient's friends and family should be advised not to discuss the patient's weight, or their own weight or weight changes, with the patient or in side conversations. If they have concerns, suggest they speak with a provider on the team.

Encourage anyone who lives in the home to strive for a weight-neutral environment, where weight and weight changes are simply not a topic of conversation.

Meal Planning

After months or years of malnutrition and emotional distress around food, nutritional rehabilitation is a daunting task. Eating in response to internal hunger and satiety cues is a long-term goal that not everyone will achieve. Anxiety about food and the stress hormones it triggers can interfere with sensations of hunger and fullness, while early satiety, delayed gastric emptying, bloating, and nausea may be misinterpreted as "fullness" or reasons to purge. Medications that impact appetite, chronic conditions, and neurodivergence can impair interoception, the bodily sensations needed to intuitively eat. So, at least for a while, nutritional rehabilitation will require assistance. Eating according to a schedule is often required to restore physical, emotional, and digestive health. This schedule is typically called a "meal plan."

No one meal planning method works for everyone. The best choice is the one that is sustainable. Whether written menus, flexible plans, or someone else preparing the food, the goal of meal planning is to support ongoing nutritional rehabilitation in a way that fits a person's learning style and literacy level; accommodates their eating preferences; adheres to special diets for medical conditions and allergies; takes into account their access to obtaining, storing, and preparing food; balances their need for structure with their desire for independence; and so on.

In a specialty care program, there is usually one preferred meal planning method that is taught to all patients. To continue the same method after discharge, each patient will need the RDN's help preparing a menu and shopping list, instruction on food preparation and plating, plus opportunities to practice before discharge. If home life is not conducive to this method, the patient will need help from the facility RDN to determine how to maintain their nutrition using a different method, and ongoing follow-up with an outpatient RDN. At the very least, a patient who is being discharged should have at least 3 days of specific menus and a grocery shopping list for those meals.

In the outpatient setting, RDNs work with each person to craft a suitable meal planning method or carry on with the method learned elsewhere. Together, the patient and RDN work out the kinks and plan for schedule changes. Within each method, the RDN has latitude to be more or less directive in providing recommendations, depending on what each patient needs and wants, and with the possibility of allowing more independence over time. As each individual gains confidence and comfort with varied eating settings, situations, and foods, structure can be decreased at their own pace. Box 6.1 lists some examples of commonly used meal-planning systems.[1-4]

BOX 6.1 Examples of Meal Planning Methods[1-4]

Meal delivery

Basic description

Fully prepared or "heat and eat" meals delivered by Meals on Wheels or other community organization, hired chef, restaurant, or outside delivery service

Best for

Someone with limited food preparation ability, executive functioning difficulty, limited mobility, or adequate food storage capacity

Limitations

Private chef service or daily restaurant delivery may be financially unrealistic for many; community services may not offer selections that meet food preferences

Daily menus

Basic description

Registered dietitian nutritionist (RDN)/patient plan exactly what will be served at each eating opportunity

Best for

Someone who struggles with making decisions in the moment, has a limited budget for food, or wants to avoid food waste

Limitations

No flexibility, spontaneity, or ability to manage unexpected situations or accept social invitations

Continued on next page

BOX 6.1 Examples of Meal Planning Methods[1-4] (cont.)

Meal schedule

Basic description

RDN/patient choose daily meal and snack times only; patient chooses from available foods at each eating opportunity

Best for

Someone with good understanding of nutrition basics who does not have a perfectionistic stance about food and can adapt as needed to what is available

Limitations

Requires a predictable daily routine and the ability to follow a schedule, set and respond to alarms

Can provoke distressing worries about making "the right choice"

Exchange plan[a,1]

Basic description

RDN determines appropriate exchange pattern at each meal

Best for

Someone who can understand and follow the exchange pattern and philosophy and who will not always choose the lowest-calorie food

Limitations

Challenging to adapt to ethnic and cultural foods, requires high literacy level

Food groups

Basic description

RDN provides daily food group goals but does not specify when to eat them

Best for

Someone who can self-regulate throughout the day so that they do not end up having to eat all their food in the evening

Limitations

Not appropriate for someone who forgets to eat or who will procrastinate without set times to eat

BOX 6.1 Examples of Meal Planning Methods[1-4] (cont.)

Calorie counting[b]

Basic description

RDN provides daily or meal-by-meal calorie goals

Best for

Someone who is already counting calories

Limitations

Not recommended in other situations

Carbohydrate counting

Basic description

RDN provides meal-by-meal grams of carbohydrate goals

Best for

Someone with type 1 diabetes

Limitations

Not recommended in other situations

The plate-by-plate approach[2]

Basic description

RDN determines which portion of a standard plate should contain which types of food

Best for

A visual learner; someone who often eats away from home or needs flexibility

Limitations

Can be manipulated if the patient always chooses the lowest-calorie options

Rule of threes[3]

Basic description

RDN educates about food groupings, including "fun food" required at lunch and dinner

Best for

Someone who appreciates specific guidelines but also likes flexible choices

Limitations

Can be manipulated if the patient always chooses the lowest-calorie options

Continued on next page

BOX 6.1 Examples of Meal Planning Methods[1-4] (cont.)

Modified family-based treatment[c]

Basic description

RDN coaches parent/caregiver to meal plan for their child

Best for

Someone with a supportive home environment and willing parents/caregivers whose food philosophy fits with recovery.

Limitation

Requires parent/caregiver availability at all mealtimes; can cause family conflict

Intuitive eating[d,4]

Basic description

Ten-step process that can include planned and unplanned eating opportunities based on a combination of internal cues, self-compassion, and "gentle" nutrition

Best for

Someone whose eating dysfunction takes the form of chronic dieting and is willing to put in the work to reconnect with the mind and body

Limitations

Can be willfully misunderstood, eg, "I wasn't hungry, so I didn't eat"; requires ability to identify emotions and internal cues such as hunger and satiety

[a] The Exchange Lists for Meal Planning were devised by a joint committee of the American Diabetes Association and the American Dietetic Association (now The Academy of Nutrition and Dietetics) to provide a universal system for the nutrition management of diabetes. "Exchanges" has now become a generic term for meal planning based on food groups. There is no standard Exchange List for eating disorder care.

[b] Although RDNs and other staff may use calorie counting as a tool for meal planning, nutrition assessment, and monitoring, it is not recommended as a nutrition education topic. One common symptom of many eating disorders is obsessive thoughts about numbers, and teaching calorie counting as a meal planning method runs the risk of creating new obsessions. If a patient is already counting calories, an individual decision should be made by the RDN, patient, and support partners, if applicable, whether to use a different meal-planning technique or whether to make use of the patient's existing calorie knowledge to support recovery.

[c] Family-based treatment historically did not include consultation with an RDN; however, the need for nutrition guidance is now recognized and RDNs are included and even lead this type of care.

[d] "Intuitive eating" was coined by Tribole and Resch to describe the 10 steps outlined in their original 1995 book. As the term has become widely used, it is often misinterpreted or considered synonymous with exclusively spontaneous eating in the absence of a meal plan, which is not accurate.

Because a long-term goal of eating recovery is more flexibility and less rigidity with food, it may seem that providing a patient with a structured meal plan is counterproductive. It is true that some patients can make a balanced meal plan seem like a new version of their eating disorder, but an RDN-devised meal plan is not intended to be a restrictive diet, and ongoing education can make this clear. The five essential differences between a recovery meal plan and a "diet" are summarized in Box 6.2.

BOX 6.2 How a Recovery Meal Plan Is Unlike a Weight-Loss Diet

A recovery meal plan is devised to promote physical and mental health, not to destroy health in search of weight loss at any cost.

A recovery meal plan is (ultimately) intended to provide adequate calories, rather than calorie deprivation, which is the goal of all weight-loss diets. Adequate caloric intake does not trigger the starvation mechanisms and eating-disordered responses that weight-loss diets cause.

A recovery meal plan is individualized (in nutrition, in format, in schedule) to meet the needs of each patient. Even though a care facility's general meal plan protocol may be the starting point, unlike weight-loss diets that are standard for everyone, a recovery meal plan will ultimately be unique for each person.

A recovery meal plan is modifiable, with input from the patient. Unlike rigid weight-loss diets that require someone to meet the same calorie goals with the same allowed foods and the same disallowed foods week after week, a recovery meal plan will be adapted on a daily, weekly, or other basis, based on the patient's changing (and hopefully improving) sense of taste, satiety, activity level, and other needs and desires.

Eventually, a recovery meal plan becomes obsolete. It is simply a tool to teach the principles of nutrition until the ability for self-nourishment returns. This is unlike weight-loss diets that tout themselves as "a lifestyle" that requires constant participation and purchases.

Internal Cues and Intuitive Eating

As nutrition status stabilizes, the roles of the patient and dietitian will progress into different stages. Depending on a patient's abilities and desire, education about identifying hunger cues while still following the meal plan may be the logical next step. Over time, the patient may take more responsibility for choosing what, when, and how much to eat. The dietitian can still provide oversight and advice while encouraging the patient to trust in their choices. And even a patient who is mostly reliant on internal cues may benefit from more direction at stressful times or when schedules change.

There is no standard or way to predict how long it will take for internal cues to normalize or to ensure that they will be reliable when they do. Research on appetite-related hormones such as leptin, ghrelin, cholecystokinin, adiponectin, insulin, and others, may add to our knowledge in this area. Notably, the term "intuitive eating" can be understood to mean anything from the 10 steps of Tribole and Resch's *Intuitive Eating* book[4] to colloquial shorthand for "eat whatever you want." It is important to define how each person is using the term.

Food Procurement and Preparation

The RDN plays a crucial role in assessing each person's skill, ability, and comfort level in obtaining and preparing food to support their recovery. The eating disorder thought process has different results for different people. Some may prefer not to interact with food at all, avoiding grocery shopping, food preparation, and even sharing space with food. Others may lack the financial resources to obtain food or food preparation skills, while others are very proficient in the kitchen, cooking and baking food for others while they refuse to nourish themselves.

Barriers to home food preparation can range from "I don't know what to buy" to "I don't want anyone at the grocery store to know I eat." Every barrier has an alternative, with the one exception of "I just don't want to." If a patient is not willing to prepare their own food, then the timing simply is not right. There are other ways to stay nourished without having to learn to cook.

Nutrition education can include everything from making a shopping list from a recipe to ordering food online, in-store grocery shopping, procuring and learning to use needed kitchen tools and supplies, learning to follow a recipe and safely use appliances, food safety and storage and preparation techniques, to how to adapt a kitchen environment to accommodate a patient's disability. The hope is that ultimately each person can advance to as much independence in eating as possible, with goals tailored to each situation.

Experiential activities that allow patients to encounter food outside of the treatment setting take nutrition education from abstract to practical, even when they do not involve the actual consumption of food. Purchasing, smelling, considering, and touching food, as well as observing others eating food, are all encounters. Grocery shopping and cooking with a dietitian, individually or in a group, can help decrease the anxiety threshold that makes these activities so intimidating.

Expert Insight

A support person struggling to understand their loved one's eating disorder may find this kind of step-by-step nutrition education unnecessarily basic, detailed, or even insulting. Help them remember that an eating disorder keeps a person from functioning at their full potential. Falling asleep after binge eating while a pot of water boils over on the stove or accidentally cross-contaminating utensils are potentially dangerous scenarios that can easily occur unless strategies are in place to prevent them.

Principles of Nutrition

In the early stages of eating disorder recovery, food rules and fears may be firmly entrenched, and meal planning may be limited to a small number of accepted foods. In high-support levels of care, challenges can be more frequent, but in the lower-support levels, increasing and advancing food intake may be much slower, wearing on both the individual and their support partners. Using the basic principles of nutrition to show that there is a planned progression of improvement can help, especially when there is frustration with the slow pace of change.

In eating disorder care, these principles are steps that build on each other, one at a time, and in a specific order, starting with priorities and moving into challenges. When adopted sequentially, they provide a solid foundation for long-term recovery. Figure 6.1 describes the principles of nutrition restoration for eating disorder recovery.

Nutritional Content of Food

As mentioned previously, education about the nutrition content of food can be misinterpreted by eating disorder thought processes and become an obsession. It can feel odd to an RDN to encourage someone to focus *less* on the nutrient content of their choices, but that is important for someone who has been attributing far too much power to individual foods or ingredients. Nutrition education in this context should include the messages that "good nutrition" is not defined or "ruined" by one food or meal, is not a guarantee of health or longevity, and is impacted by far more than just individual choices. Although this way of thinking can be disappointing to someone who thought they could control the course of their life with nutrition, it is also more realistic.

Some people who label foods as "bad" or "unhealthy" are able to completely avoid those foods and lead happy, healthy lives. But those with eating disorders either avoid so many foods that they become malnourished or experience significant distress when they eat a "bad" choice. Even worse—according to the eating disorder thought process—they may feel shame and guilt not just for eating the food but, additionally, for enjoying it.

FIGURE 6.1 Principles of nutrition restoration for eating disorder recovery

	Principle	Critera for Progression to Next Principle
Rehabilitation	Adequacy	Intake of food plus supplements meets energy needs of daily living and nutrient restoration. May rely on supplementation to meet macronutrient and micronutrient needs.
	Balance	Intake of food meets macronutrient needs of daily living. Supplementation may be used to meet additional energy needs of nutritional restoration and voluntary physical activities, or due to voluntary food exclusions.
	Variety	Intake includes several/many/most (as applicable) choices from all food groups. May include micronutrient supplementation as needed due to special needs or medically necessary food exclusions.
Education	Moderation	Intake does not exceed recommended quantities of any food, beverage, nutrient, or non-nutritive substance.
	Nutrient Density	Intake is primarily (not exclusively) composed of nutrient-rich foods. Reliance on micronutrient supplementation is limited to specific circumstances.
	Energy Balance	Energy intake meets recommendations. Nutritional supplements are used as needed, but not as a significant daily source of fuel.
Exploration	Autonomy	Intake is based on personal preferences and self-knowledge of nutrition needs rather than fear or harmful beliefs about food. Regret after eating is manageable and does not result in compensatory behaviors.
	Confidence	Intake is spontaneous and based on internal cues rather than a fixed schedule or pre-planning. Choices are almost always made without regret. No compensatory behaviors are used.

Adapted with permission from reference 5: Setnick J. Eating Disorders Boot Camp: Training Workshop for Healthcare Professionals. Accessed July 2, 2024. www.EatingDisordersBootCamp.com

> ### *Expert Insight*
>
> *Some individuals may fear reaching the confidence stage noted in Figure 6.1 on page 137 because they equate it with "losing control." The confidence stage actually represents stepping away from being controlled by food and instead exercising freedom of choice. Confidence in eating means using internal and external factors (such as hunger level, food availability, preference, and environment) to make decisions, rather than fear. The confidence level also takes into account nuance and context, so that an individual can make choices (such as declining dessert or having salad dressing on the side) that formerly would have been considered eating disorder rules. In the recovery mindset, these are simply preferences or decisions made because they are suitable to the occasion.*

"Legalizing food" describes the process of returning food to its status as simply (but so importantly) nourishment for life. It does not mean that a person will eat every food; the goal is that they will no longer feel compelled or guilty around food and will be able to make a conscious choice whether to eat it.

Rather than referring to food as "good" and "bad," useful alternatives are

- "more nutritious" or "less nutritious"
- "more to my liking" or "less to my liking"

- "unsupportive to my recovery" or "supportive to my recovery"
- or any other descriptor without a moral connotation.

Eating disorders can develop after a medical diagnosis that requires a special diet or avoidance of certain foods. When a patient has been diagnosed with a food allergy, celiac disease, diabetes, or another condition, nutrition education should of course focus on understanding what is "safe" and "unsafe" or "allowed" or "not allowed," while at the same time discouraging excessive or unnecessary restrictions and moral judgments that could compromise eating disorder recovery.

Individuals who have restricted themselves from eating some or many foods may need to relearn which foods they actually like and dislike. Recovery presents an opportunity to reevaluate food and beverage preferences and to trial different things and determine which to include in daily life, which to include only occasionally, and which to primarily avoid.

Although nutritional rehabilitation may require some challenges and discomfort, ultimately recovery does not require that a person eat or like every food. The important distinction between an appropriate food restriction and a dysfunctional one is the conscious, purposeful way the decision is made vs an impulsive, compulsive, or reactionary manner. Ideally, the motive for each eating choice is individually determined, rather than based on the perceptions of others, mistaken beliefs, or shame.

Nutrition Needs of Activity

Physical activity guidelines for an individual with an eating disorder should be made by the treatment team based on the patient's physical stability and health, current nutrition intake, and past history of exercise compulsivity. Education about the energy cost of daily living, additional needs of activity, and how to adapt the meal plan may be needed.

Someone who has used exercise as a purging method, or who has competed but never experienced leisurely exercise, may benefit from guidance about which types of exercise are appropriate at each stage of recovery, including noncompetitive, social, or meditative forms of exercise like yoga, dancing for fun, or leisure walks. Competition and team sports should be avoided until much later in recovery, as patients may find it difficult to respect their physical limitations or respond to signs of fatigue when competing or when they think others are relying on their performance.

> **_Expert Insight_**
>
> *If a patient is unable to meet their daily energy needs or the additional needs of exercise, voluntary activities should be restricted. Just because a patient has been "medically cleared" to exercise does not mean they are nutritionally ready.*

Harmful Behaviors

Education regarding the harmful effects of eating disorder behaviors is not usually effective at changing them. Skipping meals, binge eating, vomiting, laxative use, and self-harm may have compulsive aspects, even self-soothing features. Nutrition education will usually be more productive if it focuses on facts and practicalities rather than dangers.

In the case of laxatives, this might include an explanation of the normal process of digestion and the length of time that food normally takes to travel through the digestive tract, along with asking a support person to remove laxatives from a patient's home.

For binge eating, a useful topic is the restrict-binge cycle. Patients often think of undereating as a goal and binge eating as a failure. Hearing a dietitian connect the two can help a patient recognize that restrictive eating is in fact driving their binge behavior.

With regard to self-induced vomiting, asking for support after mealtimes or brainstorming distracting activities can be useful.

Restaurants and Social Eating Settings

Nutrition education can address how to maintain eating recovery in social eating settings and other situations where an individual is not able to prepare their own food. The RDN and patient should address the most likely scenarios first, such as practicing reviewing a restaurant menu in advance, asking about special dietary requests when needed, and autonomy when others offer unwanted food. An especially important area for education is how to maintain boundaries when eating companions talk about food or discuss their own eating practices. Real-world recovery requires the ability to ignore or walk away from unhelpful discussions about food and eating.

Some social situations are less predictable and more stressful—even without the added stress of the eating aspect—such as a first date, meeting a significant other's parents, or participating in a wedding, performance, or reunion. In extremely stressful or hostile social situations, it may be best for an individual to plan not to eat at the event at all. In that case, the RDN can help modify the meal plan for the times before and after the event. Body image issues can flare up around this type of event, and alcohol may be present, so an individual who struggles with either or both of these may benefit from additional support and planning from a mental health professional.

Summary of Nutrition Education in Eating Disorders

As with all nutrition interventions for eating disorders, the nutrition education provided by an RDN will vary extensively from patient to patient and from setting to setting. In a brief hospital stay for crisis stabilization, nutrition education may be a low priority compared with medical care, and an RDN may only have one chance to meet with a patient. The best use of this time may be in explaining the basics of the RDN role in assisting with nutrition and eating disorder recovery and offering a referral to an outpatient dietitian.

If the hospital stay is long enough for multiple visits, address the patient's harmful beliefs about food and focus on small, practical steps they can take after discharge to improve their nutritional status. Education in acute care may not result in long-term change. Even if a patient eats while hospitalized, their eating disorder has not been cured.

Providing education to a patient's family members and support partners can be especially helpful when it helps them understand their loved one's condition and what may be expected of them after discharge, such as food shopping and supporting the patient at mealtimes. They may welcome information and having someone to answer their questions, recommend reading materials, and local or online caregiver support groups.

If there is no eating disorder specialty facility available to meet a patient's needs, or a patient is primarily in the hospital for a medical illness and during that stay an eating disorder is diagnosed, they may remain in acute care long enough to advance their nutrition significantly and meet with a dietitian several times. When a dietitian develops a relationship with a patient over weeks or months, nutrition education can be more effective as the patient is better nourished, able to think more clearly, and more trusting of the dietitian's point of view.

Eating disorder treatment programs often have their own nutrition education curriculum, usually provided in a group setting. Lectures like "Why You Need Carbs" or "Talking About Healthy Fats" can be ineffective and even harmful. Nutrition education is far better when it is related to the true experience of eating disorder treatment and recovery, such as "How to Avoid Comparing Plates" or "How to Navigate a Buffet." These are practical topics from which interaction and discussion can be tailored to the needs of the individuals present. Cooking classes, grocery tours, restaurant meals, and other experiences are also worthwhile nutrition education tools.

Nutrition education is also crucially important for a patient's support partners, especially those who will be taking responsibility for meal preparation after discharge. Giving them the same information and predicting and problem-solving stressful situations can minimize disagreements over nutrient content, portion sizes, and anything else that will distract from the patient's recovery.

The vast majority of comprehensive nutrition education will be provided in conjunction with outpatient nutrition counseling. With the luxury of time, nutrition education topics can be introduced gradually, repeatedly, and in the context of a patient's daily challenges. Teaching the practical steps of consistent, daily eating opportunities; obtaining, safely storing, and preparing food; and other real-world topics will advance recovery better than nutrition science or a generic curriculum given to all patients.

More nutrition information is not better if the information is distorted or misunderstood. To be effective, nutrition education should be interactive, with opportunities to ask questions about the new information, consider how it counteracts currently held beliefs, and discuss how it can be applied to each patient's life. This includes adapting information to family members and other support partners who will be taking part in the eating or food preparation process for or with the patient.

The importance of including supportive individuals cannot be overstated. In many cases, the family *is* the treatment team, dedicating themselves to their loved one's recovery. Eating disorders cause collateral damage far beyond the patient, and assisting support partners in their own emotional recovery is in the realm of the mental health providers. But nutrition education and counseling sessions are a golden opportunity to find out how the nutrition plan can be strengthened and refined from the people who are actually implementing it. They have been hurt by their loved one's condition and should be included in the healing process, too. Incorporating the individuals who support each patient and helping them with their questions and concerns ultimately benefits everyone.

References

1. Holler HJ. Understanding the use of the exchange lists for meal planning in diabetes management. *Diabetes Educ.* 1991;17(6):474-484. doi:10.1177/014572179101700611
2. Crosbie C, Sterling W. *How to Nourish Yourself Through an Eating Disorder: Recovery for Adults With the Plate-by-Plate Approach.* The Experiment; 2023.
3. Herrin M, Larkin M. *Nutrition Counseling in the Treatment of Eating Disorders.* 2nd ed. Taylor & Francis Group; 2013.
4. Tribole E, Resch E. *Intuitive Eating.* 4th ed. St. Martin's Essentials; 2020.
5. Setnick J. Eating Disorders Boot Camp: Training Workshop for Healthcare Professionals. Accessed July 2, 2024. www.eatingdisordersbootcamp.com

CHAPTER 7

Nutrition Intervention for Eating Disorders: Nutrition Counseling

Nutrition counseling is an ongoing conversation about nutrition, food, eating, and related topics. Nutrition counseling is interwoven with nutrition assessment, nutrition education, and food and nutrient delivery. Nutrition counseling is a collaboration between the registered dietitian nutritionist (RDN) and patient that may make use of therapeutic techniques. However, nutrition counseling is not psychotherapy or mental health counseling.

Dietitians who specialize in eating disorders are often included under the umbrella of mental health professionals simply by working in the mental health field. But our dietitian credentials and the topics that we approach differentiate us from mental health counselors. Many dietitians worry that we are stepping outside the scope of appropriate practice when we feel like we are "having a conversation" with a patient. This comes from a misunderstanding—the idea that nutrition counseling requires an authoritative tone rather than a mutually respectful relationship. A friendly dietitian or a joking conversation are not signs that nutrition counseling has gone off track; they are simply the way that people communicate. Familiarity, kindness, and even humor can be great assets in the process of change, as a patient is more likely to listen when being treated as an equal and given the opportunity to participate in their own care.

At the same time, boundaries between patient and dietitian are crucially important. We must not burden patients with our personal stress, workplace issues, or anything else unrelated to their care. We do not socialize with them, or set them up on dates, or violate their privacy when we see them elsewhere. We set the tone for our sessions by being on time, acknowledging our mistakes, and directing the conversation toward the topic at hand.

In a secure, ongoing nutrition counseling relationship, conversations flow toward and away from nutrition-related topics. What people do and think about their food and bodies are very personal topics, so when coming in from the outside world, a patient may need time to transition from small talk to serious business. If small talk or "How was your week?" responses start to take up too much of your allotted time, validate the importance of the event to the patient, and then use a transitional phrase to move the topic on to nutrition. For example:

- "That's so interesting! ... I'm curious how that affected your eating."
- "I'm so glad you had that experience! ... Tell me—did it make a difference in your eating?"
- "That does sound like a great weekend! ... Do you think your eating disorder played a role in how it turned out?"

And if your attempts at transitioning gently are not effective:

- "I've enjoyed hearing about that (or I'm sorry to hear about that). ... I would like to hear more, but I'm concerned that we won't have time left for what we need to cover if we don't switch to talking about nutrition now."

Chapter 7

The Intersecting Roles of Dietitian and Therapist

Conversations about bodies, weight, food, and eating occur in both dietitian and therapist sessions. They are complex issues in a society that portrays body size and appearance as intrinsically related to happiness, relationships, safety, and love. They may require more sifting to find a nutrition component. And if we determine that an issue is not related to eating at all, we can simply say, "I'm so glad you mentioned that, it seems really important, but I'm not the best person to advise you." Being human is never out of our scope.

One of our strengths as dietitians is knowing what food and nutrition can and cannot do. We sift through a patient's situation to find aspects that nutrition counseling can address. Many situations seemingly not about food on the surface have some connection to nutrition or eating, especially for an individual working to heal from an eating disorder. We can often find a nutrition angle or topic by gently asking a question. "Do you think that's related to your eating disorder?" or "How do you think that affected your eating?" are useful when we are not sure.

Of course, there are topics that genuinely do not relate to eating or nutrition no matter how deep a dietitian looks, and others where, in addition to nutritional counseling, additional help is needed. Relationship drama, adverse childhood experiences, upcoming life changes, just to name a few, may benefit from a different type of care.

A patient may seek the services of an RDN thinking that their issues have roots in nutrition, not realizing there is more to the picture. The RDN may be the very first person in whom a patient has confided. In these cases, a sensitive and caring referral to a mental health professional is a gift. If the topic comes up again, the RDN can simply say, "That seems important, but I'm not the right person to advise you."

Overview of Counseling Techniques

The beauty of nutrition counseling is that it does not require adherence to one specific modality or counseling theory but can pull pertinent concepts from multiple sources to craft the most useful tools for each individual's needs. This section reviews some specific counseling theories you may encounter in eating disorder care. Not all are appropriate for every patient or situation, specifically neurodiverse individuals and those with past bad experiences related to a certain modality. The art of nutrition counseling is a blend of knowledge—matching the technique to each person and situation—and flexibility—changing direction when needed.

Motivational Interviewing

The success of nutrition counseling relies on each individual patient's willingness to work toward recovery, confidence that change is achievable, and ability to persevere in the face of difficulties that will no doubt arise. This is often described as readiness for change, part of the transtheoretical model.[1]

Motivational interviewing (MI) assesses and attempts to improve motivation to change and opens the door to action.[2] MI techniques include active and reflective listening, open-ended questions, affirmation, and summarization, all of which are appropriate in nutrition counseling. MI also includes discussing ambivalence and reluctance to change.

Cognitive Behavioral Therapy*

Cognitive behavioral therapy (CBT) is based on the concept that behaviors (the way we think is considered a behavior) are learned and can be unlearned with practice.[3,4] It takes a long time to change thought patterns,

* Note a difference between CBT and enhanced CBT (CBT-E): CBT-E is a specific, time-limited, manualized treatment model. It relies exclusively on treatment by psychotherapists without consultation with dietitians. Easily confused due to similar names and acronyms, CBT is a treatment theory that can be adapted to nutrition counseling, while CBT-E is a treatment model.

but someone in danger does not have the luxury of that time. When they eat, even though they are not mentally "ready," they will experience negative feelings. In order to press onward (rather than returning to harmful behaviors), they will need alternative ways to feel better. Called "coping skills," these alternatives (ie, different ways of thinking, feeling, and acting) are the goal of CBT.

Planning ahead, problem solving, role playing imaginary situations, legalizing food, keeping a list of supportive activities and people, and identifying the thoughts and feelings that drive eating behavior are all ways RDNs use CBT principles.

Dialectical Behavior Therapy

Dialectical behavior therapy (DBT) was developed by Marsha Linehan, PhD, ABPP, to help individuals with self-harming and suicidal behaviors identify their destructive thoughts without acting on them.[5] DBT is taught in many eating disorder treatment settings as a way to interrupt the path from thoughts to behaviors.

A foundational principle of DBT is that the counselor nonjudgmentally accepts the patient's thoughts and feelings while pointing out other options. This is an easy fit for RDNs who always attempt to align with a patient in a nonjudgmental manner, identify multiple possibilities for how to reach a goal, and assist the patient in determining which method to try.

The four core strategies of DBT are mindfulness, distress tolerance, emotion regulation, and interpersonal effectiveness. When emotion regulation and interpersonal effectiveness skills are taught by a mental health professional, the RDN can suggest eating situations in which to use them. Many RDNs teach mindfulness and distress tolerance concepts, sometimes without calling them those names, because they come naturally in conversations about eating. *Mindfulness* may include learning to listen for and identifying physical sensations of hunger and satiety, cravings, and the nonhunger feelings that trigger eating behaviors. *Distress tolerance* may include learning to acknowledge the desire to use a compensatory behavior and using an alternate behavior to manage it.

Acceptance and Commitment Therapy

Acceptance and commitment therapy (ACT) is an offshoot of DBT that can be applied to eating disorder treatment. ACT strategies that are useful for dietitians include defusing (separating thoughts from reality), identifying values for life, and committing to using values to determine the best course of action.[6]

Family-Based Treatment

Family-based treatment is not a counseling theory but a manualized treatment methodology.[7] It was groundbreaking in the psychotherapy field because it included family members in eating disorder treatment for the first time. It was not groundbreaking for dietitians for two reasons:

1. Dietitians have always looked to family members, when available, to support patients.
2. The original iterations of FBT specifically excluded dietitians from participating.

FBT has more recently been adapted to include dietitians and to provide a more comprehensive approach to treatment.

Emotion-Focused Family Therapy

Emotion-focused family therapy (EFFT) was developed by Adele Lafrance, PhD, as a way to help an entire family rather than focusing on one person.[8] Dietitians who specialize in eating disorder care have found the principles of EFFT to be very helpful in defusing volatile family situations and helping caregivers align around their child's best interests.

Internal Family Systems

The concept of internal family systems (IFS) was founded by Richard Schwartz, PhD, as a way to nonjudgmentally identify each person's multiple points of view into "parts."[9] This allows a person to be ambivalent about change without requiring one "part" to be right or wrong; to have conversations among the parts; and to acknowledge that all of the parts have a role in keeping the person safe. Many dietitians have found IFS to be extremely conducive to eating disorder nutrition counseling as it allows each patient to choose their own values and make choices based on safety rather than fear.

Other Counseling Techniques and Modalities

Nutrition counseling for eating disorders may include aspects of other counseling techniques and modalities depending on an individual dietitian's training and expertise. Dozens of different kinds of therapeutic techniques are used in eating disorder treatment: rational emotive behavior theory, radically open dialectical behavior therapy, emotion acceptance behavior therapy, cognitive remediation therapy, family systems theory, eye movement desensitization therapy, bio- and neurofeedback, brainspotting, exposure and response prevention, integrative cognitive-affective therapy, eagala and equine-assisted psychotherapy, massage therapy, and expressive therapies including art, music, dance, and psychodrama, among many others. In addition, modalities from indigenous and nonwestern cultures exist that can add ancient wisdom to the mix: mutual aid, acupuncture, Ayurveda, yoga, psilocybin, and other psychedelics, just to name a few.

Mainstream eating disorder research and treatment has historically been gatekept, academic, and focused on a very narrow patient profile. As the eating disorder field wakes up to its own closed-mindedness and enters an era of recognition that healing comes in many forms, a wider variety of modalities are being recognized. Because there is no "standard" eating disorder patient, there is no standard treatment we can expect to benefit everyone.

RDNs do not necessarily practice these therapies and modalities; in many cases, they require special training, credentials, and equipment. But we are excellent at individualizing care and helping our patients find the methods and modalities that suit them best. And as an eclectic form of therapy, nutrition counseling can pull from a variety of sources to facilitate behavior change and healing.

Appendix D contains a list of additional books and resources by and for RDNs that teach counseling skills useful in eating disorder care.

References

1. Weiss CV, Mills JS, Westra HA, Carter JC. A preliminary study of motivational interviewing as a prelude to intensive treatment for an eating disorder. *J Eat Disord*. 2013;1:34. doi:10.1186/2050-2974-1-34
2. Spahn JM, Reeves RS, Keim KS, et al. State of the evidence regarding behavior change theories and strategies in nutrition counseling to facilitate health and food behavior change.*J Am Diet Assoc*. 2010;110(6):879-891. doi:10.1016/j.jada.2010.03.021
3. Kleifield EI, Wagner S, Halmi KA. Cognitive-behavioral treatment of anorexia nervosa. *Psychiatr Clin North Am*. 1996;19(4):715-737. doi:10.1016/s0193-953x(05)70377-4
4. Baldwin TT, Falciglia GA. Application of cognitive behavioral theories to dietary change in clients.*J Am Diet Assoc*. 1995;95(11):1315-1317. doi:10.1016/S0002-8223(95)00344-4
5. Linehan M. *DBT Skills Training Manual*. 2nd ed. Guilford Press; 2014.
6. Dindo L, Van Liew JR, Arch JJ. Acceptance and commitment therapy: a transdiagnostic behavioral intervention for mental health and medical conditions. *Neurotherapeutics*. 2017;14(3):546-553. doi:10.1007/s13311-017-0521-3
7. Rienecke RD, Le Grange D. The five tenets of family-based treatment for adolescent eating disorders.*J Eat Disord*. 2022;10(1):60. doi:10.1186/s40337-022-00585-y
8. Robinson AL, Dolhanty J, Greenberg L. Emotion-focused family therapy for eating disorders in children and adolescents. *Clin Psychol Psychother*. 2015;22(1):75-82. doi:10.1002/cpp.1861
9. Schwartz RC, Sweezy M. *Internal Family Systems Therapy*. 2nd ed. Guilford Press; 2019.

CHAPTER 8

Nutrition Intervention for Eating Disorders: Coordination of Care

Coordination of care, or referring a patient to other resources, becomes part of the registered dietitian nutritionist's (RDN's) role when we inform other providers of our findings, consult with other disciplines, and recommend a patient seeks additional types of care. In eating disorder treatment facilities where a team of professionals has an appropriate caseload and works well together, coordination and patient care may run smoothly. In facilities with high turnover, inexperienced staff, or poor leadership, care coordination—and patient care—will suffer.

In a general hospital without eating disorder specialists, care coordination often resides with a case manager or social worker who can identify options in the community and set up appointments on a patient's behalf. In an outpatient setting, college campus, or private practice, the RDN may be the person making those connections for a patient. Regardless of where eating disorder care takes place, a variety of disciplines will each have a role. The providers, the patient, and the patient's support partners all comprise the eating disorder treatment team, and attempts should be made to include all members in major treatment decisions.

Types of Care Coordination

Coordinating Medical Care

Malnutrition, the common thread of all eating disorders, affects every bodily function, organ system, and mental process. Eating disorder treatment always requires medical care, mental health care, and nutritional rehabilitation, but often that is not enough. At any given time, an individual experiencing an eating disorder might have any number of pressing physical, mental, and emotional issues. Sadly, most individuals experiencing eating disorders get no treatment at all. Some are offered standard care for the most pressing issue without anyone addressing the underlying factors, but relatively few receive comprehensive, eating disorder-informed care.

Identification, assessment, and treatment of eating disorders are topics not covered in the education or training of most physicians or health professionals, including dietitians.[1-3] Simply by reading this book, you may be the most eating disorder-aware provider on your patient's treatment team. And when you are the first provider to identify a problem, you may be the first person to alert your patient of the need to assemble a team.

Everything from insurance changes and other transitions, houselessness, geography, work and family responsibilities, disability, poverty, and scarcity of providers can contribute to situations in which an individual with an eating disorder does not have a stable source of medical care. Even for those with insurance and access, specialists (or even knowledgeable generalists) are frustratingly rare. Instead of the ideal (each patient has access to an eating disorder-informed medical provider who is updated and able to regularly follow them), we can often only hope for a well-meaning general medical provider a patient can turn to when needed.

The technicalities of communicating with other care providers will of course depend on the care setting. In a facility or hospital, permission to share protected health information and communicate with outside providers (sometimes called a "release of information") may already have been obtained during the admission process. In a private practice setting, the dietitian or office staff may gather permission to communicate with and release information to a patient's other care providers.

The best time to share information is right away. If there is no established method of communication, such as patient care rounds or staffing meetings, it will be up to each RDN to establish a method of communication with the patient's other providers. Reaching out after the first meeting with a new patient ensures that the other providers are aware the patient is receiving medical nutrition therapy and that they have the opportunity to share their concerns. The format for each communication will depend on what the providers have established in advance and the urgency of each situation. For dietitians in outpatient care, especially those working virtually or in nonhospital settings, the ability to quickly reach a patient's medical provider (or their office) can be a crucially important safety issue.

As treatment proceeds, the frequency of communication may change depending on whether difficulties develop, the patient's condition improves, or additional referrals are needed. It is important to document whenever communication takes place.

Expert Insight

When a patient or family member reports something irregular that another provider said or did, double-check the situation with the other provider to clarify what took place. In times of crisis, the chance of misinterpretation or misunderstanding is high, and both the patient and the other provider deserve the courtesy of clarification.

Coordinating Mental Health Care

Mental health care has many forms, names, and provider types. Licensed mental health providers in a given state may include psychologists, behavioral or advanced practice nurses, social workers, marriage and family therapists, professional counselors, guidance counselors, chaplains, and others. Psychiatrists may provide a combination of medical and mental health care or specialize in one or the other.

As with dietitians, the mental health field encompasses a wide range of eating disorder expertise and specialties. (Refer to Chapter 7 for a description of counseling techniques used in eating disorder treatment.) Some familiarity with eating disorder treatment can be helpful, but specialization may be less important than a personality and philosophy that match with the patient. A willingness to coordinate with the dietitian is, of course, ideal. It may take more than one try for a patient to find a good fit.

Dietitians are generally not trained to take the lead in patient care, but we rise to the situation when we identify a need. Because eating and eating problems are obviously in our realm, there is a level of comfort people feel in telling us about their difficulties with food. It is up to us to sift out, sometimes over time, whether those difficulties have a nutrition solution or ultimately rest outside our scope. Connecting a patient with mental health care is an important and often essential step in eating recovery.[4] Box 8.1 offers examples of reasons an RDN may refer a patient to mental health care.

BOX 8.1 Reasons to Refer to a Mental Health Professional

Diagnosis of psychiatric illness, including eating disorder

Relationship or family problems, recent or past

Difficulty adjusting to a recent life change

Behavior changes as a result of stress or life events

Difficulty caring for self or dependents and difficulty with activities of daily living

Traumatic event(s), including diagnosis of severe, stigmatizing, or debilitating illness and medical recommendations that change quality of life (eg, bed rest, chemotherapy, insulin shots)

Depression, anxiety, or other overwhelming emotions, whether reported or observed (eg, crying in session, agitation, pacing, anger)

Family member(s) preoccupied with patient's weight or eating

Sudden change in behavior, mood, or mental state, reported or observed

Inability to change even though patient expresses that change is desired

Fear, anxiety, stress, whether warranted or unwarranted, about the course of the eating disorder or recovery

A patient who does not immediately agree to pursue mental health care may need more information or time to reflect on the suggestion. They may think counseling is distasteful or embarrassing, something they "don't need" or "already did," or consider it a weakness or flaw. Box 8.2 lists possible reflections.

BOX 8.2 Overcoming Objections to Mental Health Care

Frame counseling as bringing another perspective onto the team: "The skills you and I bring to the table haven't been able to solve your eating. I'd like to get another point of view that could help us sort it out."

Name specific issues that could benefit from counseling: "Time management/raising teenagers/work-life balance isn't my area, but I know there are people who can really help with that."

Relate counseling to nutrition: "You've told me you feel comfortable talking with me about your eating. I'd like to help you find a counselor you feel comfortable talking to about other things."

Describe the outcome you hope for: "You and I have made so much progress on your eating. I'd love for you to feel that same way in other areas."

A counselor as a back-up plan: "Things are going well, and I'm glad, but as we move forward with your eating, we might find spots that flare up. I'd like to have a counselor in place even if you're not meeting regularly right now."

Set a time limit: "How long should we work on this before we ask a counselor for help? I'd like you to make an appointment in case we're still working on this by then."

Make a list: "I understand you're not ready to meet with a counselor. When a topic comes up that's outside of my scope, I'm going to add it to this list. That way when you're ready, we'll have this list that you can bring."

Set a boundary: "We've come to a point where continuing to meet isn't moving us forward. Rather than setting up another appointment, let's wait until you've scheduled with a counselor before we meet again."

> ***Expert Insight***
>
> *Parting ways with a patient can be painful, especially when you were hoping for a different outcome. Thoughtfully consider your options in consultation with a colleague or supervisor.*

Coordinating Additional Care

Depending on an individual's symptoms and needs, a variety of additional support may be added over the course of treatment, either for evaluation and consultation, or on an ongoing basis. RDNs are not always trained to recommend or make referrals to providers in other disciplines. We may imagine that care coordination is the job of the nurse or social worker, or that we should step back so the medical provider can take the lead. If that is the way your clinic or hospital works, that's great. Pass your recommendation up the chain. However, in private practice, outpatient care, or a facility where other providers are not eating disorder-informed, the RDN will need to fill this role. Refer when a patient would benefit from different, additional, or specialist care, or when they have a need that is out of the RDN scope of practice. If you are unsure, consult with a colleague, but do not keep silent when you see a need.

Box 8.3 on page 158 includes potential team members to whom you may refer your patients.

BOX 8.3 Supplementary Treatment Team Members

Team member	*Role*	*Reason to refer*
Art therapist	Emotional access and healing through creative expression	Difficulty with self-expression in talk therapy
Cardiologist	Cardiac care Medical clearance for physical activity	Chest pain, palpitations, shortness of breath Rapid or significant weight loss History or family history of heart disease
Dentist	Dental care	Chronic vomiting whether voluntary or not Teeth grinding Gum disease and tooth loss due to malnutrition
Endocrinologist	Hormone evaluation Insulin resistance Diabetes management	Weight change out of proportion to eating pattern Irregular or absent menstrual cycle not attributed to malnutrition Significant weight gain at menarche or menopause Infertility Symptoms of diabetes, hypoglycemia, hypothyroidism or hyperthyroidism, polycystic ovary syndrome
Family therapist	Provide support to patient in communicating and improving relationships with family members	Family members argue during or about nutrition counseling Family dynamics contribute to or perpetuate eating disorder behavior Family members not coping well with stress

BOX 8.3 Supplementary Treatment Team Members (cont.)

Team member	*Role*	*Reason to refer*
Gastroenterologist	Digestive care	Chronic vomiting or laxative abuse Vomiting Blood in stool Chronic abdominal pain Reflux Diagnosis or symptoms of celiac disease, Crohn's disease, or irritable bowel syndrome Chronic or severe constipation or diarrhea
Group therapist	Support group leader	Poor social support network Desire for peer interaction
Occupational therapist	Feeding therapy, recommendation of adaptive feeding devices, cooking tools and cooking and eating environment	Difficulty with self-feeding Difficulty with physical movements required to prepare food
Physical therapist, exercise physiologist, personal trainer, or other movement therapist	Exercise prescription Injury rehabilitation Stress management, relaxation, release of physical tension	Patient has been medically approved to exercise Patient is recovering from injury Patient unaware of appropriate intensity/duration/mode of physical activity
Psychiatrist or psychiatric nurse practitioner	Evaluation, diagnosis, medication management	Any eating disorder Anxiety Depression

Continued on next page

BOX 8.3 Supplementary Treatment Team Members (cont.)

Team member	Role	Reason to refer
Religious leader	Spiritual healing	Religious beliefs or conflict with god/higher power impairing recovery History of religious abuse (religion used as weapon of guilt or shame in childhood)
Speech therapist or speech-language pathologist	Feeding evaluation, feeding therapy, recommendation of adaptive feeding devices	Difficulty chewing or swallowing food or beverages Repeated choking Aversion to eating or swallowing

Expert Insight

If you are in contact with a patient's other providers, it is considerate to inform them that you have made a referral to another provider. If possible, contact the new team member to update them before the patient's first appointment.

Discharge and Transfer to a New Setting

There is no standard of care for when an individual patient should stop meeting with a dietitian. Some transitions are initiated by a patient when they have a life change, location change, insurance change, or simply wish to change dietitians. If a patient's condition continues to improve to the point where regular follow-up sessions are not needed, time between appointments can be extended further and further, with the option of changing the frequency if needed.

If a patient's condition continues to deteriorate, or takes a turn for the worse, their dietitian may discharge them for hospitalization or admission to a treatment program or facility. Hopefully the patient's condition will then improve enough that they can step down into decreasing levels of care and—if mutually agreed—return to that dietitian's care.

A change in care or support level ideally is made in consultation with all members of the treatment team, but that is not always possible. In cases of emergency or disagreement among providers or support partners, consensus may not be realistic or achievable. It is an unfortunate fact that insurance company representatives (who generally have never met the patient) often have the last word in determining a patient's options for care.

Levels of Care in Eating Disorder Treatment

Outpatient Care

In outpatient eating disorder care, individual appointments are made with care providers in an office or clinic setting. Patients appropriate for this level of care are:

- medically stable and in at least fair general health, requiring infrequent monitoring of weight or vital signs;
- self-motivated toward recovery and in a stable and supportive living environment;

- able to travel to and from scheduled appointments safely and reliably;
- able to follow a meal plan at home or school (100% compliance not required);
- able to resist purging, exercise, and self-harm triggers at home (100% compliance not required); and
- not actively suicidal.

Intensive Outpatient Program

In an intensive outpatient program, group meetings are supervised by care providers in 2- to 4-hour increments several times per week. Patients appropriate for this level of care are:

- medically stable and at least in fair general health but possibly requiring weight or vital signs to be monitored approximately once per week;
- self-motivated toward recovery and in a stable and supportive living environment;
- able to travel to and from group and individual meetings safely and reliably;
- able to follow a meal plan at home or school (100% compliance not required);
- able to resist purging, exercise, and self-harm triggers at home (100% compliance not required); and
- not actively suicidal.

Day Treatment

Day treatment is also called *full-day outpatient care* or *partial hospitalization*. Individual and group treatment is offered for the majority of waking hours most days of the week, including one or more supervised meals each day. Day treatment programs may operate during typical work or school hours, such as 8 AM to 4 PM, Monday through Friday.

Partial hospitalization typically refers to spending 7 days per week in a hospital treatment program, including all meals, but returning home to sleep. Patients appropriate for this level of care are:

- medically stable to leave the hospital or facility but requiring weight or vital signs to be monitored daily;
- having difficulty following a meal plan without supervision at mealtimes;
- having difficulty resisting purging or self-harm triggers without supervision;
- self-motivated enough in treatment to attempt to avoid detrimental behaviors when unsupervised at home in a stable living environment;
- able to travel to and from the facility safely and reliably; and
- not actively suicidal.

Residential Treatment or Treatment Center

Sometimes referred to as "rehab," residential treatment is conducted in a freestanding treatment facility that may or may not be affiliated with a hospital and may or may not be devoted exclusively to eating disorder care. Patients appropriate for this level of care are:

- medically compromised and requiring daily or constant monitoring of weight or vital signs;
- unable to travel safely or reliably to treatment;
- in an unstable or unsupportive living environment;
- unable to follow a meal plan without supervision and external motivation;
- unable to resist purging or self-harm triggers without supervision and external motivation and so require supervision using the bathroom; and
- resistant or uncooperative in recovery, requiring constant structure and external motivation to remain safe.

Inpatient Hospitalization

Depending on the location, 24-hour hospitalization can take different forms. An individual diagnosed with an eating disorder may be admitted to a medical floor, behavioral or psychiatric unit, or an eating disorder-specific treatment program. Guidelines from the American Psychiatric Association recommend that any patient meeting the following metrics be admitted on an inpatient basis[5]:

- medically unstable and requiring daily or constant monitoring of weight, vital signs, or laboratory tests, including:
  - heart rate less than 40 beats per minute (adult) or near 40 beats per minute (child/adolescent)
  - blood pressure less than 90/60 mm Hg (adult) or less than 80/50 mm Hg (child/adolescent)
  - Greater than 10 to 20 mm Hg drop in blood pressure from sitting to standing position
  - glucose level less than 60 mg/dL
  - potassium less than 3 mEq/L
  - temperature less than 97°F
  - dehydrated, hypokalemic, or hypophosphatemic, or experiencing hepatic, renal, or cardiovascular complications requiring acute treatment
- malnourished or refusing oral intake, possibly requiring nutrition support;
- weighing less than 85% of expected weight in adults or refusing food or experiencing acute weight loss in children, even if weight is within normal limits;
- purging or self-harming unless constantly supervised and may be actively suicidal and may secretly exercise if left unsupervised and requires supervision using the bathroom;
- resistant or uncooperative in recovery, requiring constant structure and external motivation to remain safe, actively attempting to sabotage medical/nutritional care; and
- not medically unstable but they are psychiatrically impaired or chemically dependent.

"Step-down" Care, Transitional Living, "Halfway" House, or Group Home

After leaving inpatient or residential treatment, patients may participate in a less-structured living situation intended to prepare them to return to their own home and outpatient care. This is especially important if the patient's home living situation is not stable or if the patient will be living alone for the first time.

If the inpatient or residential facility does not provide step-down care, options may be available in the patient's hometown. At this level of care, supervision varies by facility. Facilities may provide a combination of group or individual therapy, 12-step meetings, a case worker or on-site supervisor, communal meals, curfews, and drug screenings—or none of these. Some facilities are simply a safe place to live and practice recovery. A patient appropriate for this level of care will meet the standards for outpatient care with the exception of the stable home living environment, as this will be provided by the step-down facility itself.

Ideally, an individual does not switch overnight from inpatient to outpatient care but instead is able to step down to a lower level of care over time, practicing their independent living skills without being totally self-reliant. This type of transitional living is common for individuals recovering from drug or alcohol dependence but rare for those recovering from eating disorders. Depending on the community resources available, many patients seek treatment away from home and then must find local providers in their hometown. These patients often struggle with the enormity of the transition and the drastic decrease in daily support they receive.

A common misconception that contributes to this difficult adjustment is that patients discharged from inpatient or residential care are now "cured" and no longer practicing their eating disorder. The reality is that duration of treatment is often limited by health insurance providers, and many patients leave care before achieving a stable level of recovery or the ability to maintain it. In addition, home life entails higher levels of stressors of all kinds, rendering the skills obtained in the sterile environment of a treatment center far less effective. It is very common for patients to regress in their recovery in the first few weeks postdischarge. It is in the best interest of the patient to have outpatient care appointments scheduled prior to discharge so that the facility dietitian can communicate necessary and helpful information to the outpatient dietitian.

Matching a Patient to an Eating Disorder Treatment Facility

Finding an eating disorder treatment facility can be a challenging task for a patient and their support partners. Depending on their priorities, consider the following.

- Does the facility accept patients who are medically unstable?
- Does the facility provide medical care and medical nutritional rehabilitation when indicated?
- What is the facility's philosophy of treatment? Their nutrition philosophy? Their philosophy regarding eating disorders?
- Does the facility aid patients in finding follow-up care?
- What is the cost? What insurance coverage is available? Are payment plans available? Are charity beds available?
- What are criteria for discharge? What is the average length of stay?
- Is the facility only for patients with eating disorders or for all patients needing psychiatric care?
- What gender(s) does the facility serve? Do they admit transgender or gender-nonconforming patients?
- Does the facility have clinicians who share the same identity/identities as the patient?
- Does the facility allow patient food preferences? What about cultural foods similar to those the patient will eat in their home? Does the facility have a kosher kitchen or provide a halal option?
- Does the facility provide accommodations for a disabled or neurodivergent patient?
- Does the facility provide treatment for additional issues that patients may have, such as trauma, substance abuse, or self-harm?

- Are visitors allowed? Do visitors or family members participate in treatment?
- Does the facility have a particular religious affiliation?
- Does the facility offer a step-down program?

Insurance Coverage for Eating Disorders

Accessing insurance coverage for eating disorder care is often a challenge. The Paul Wellstone and Pete Domenici Mental Health Parity and Addiction Equity Act of 2008[6] (MHPAEA) made it illegal for insurers to utilize different standards for mental health and substance use benefits than they do for medical and surgical benefits. Even after the passage of MHPAEA, many patients continued to report difficulty accessing medical nutrition therapy for eating disorder care. Therefore in 2024, federal regulators clarified the MHPAEA requirements for eating disorder treatment. These "final rules"[7] state that "nutrition counseling is the primary treatment for eating disorders in the outpatient [setting]" and that "not covering nutrition counseling for the treatment of eating disorders while covering it for medical conditions" is a frank violation of the law.

Obtaining insurance coverage for eating disorder treatment is rarely straightforward and typically requires many exchanges back and forth between insurance personnel, the insured, and providers. Many issues exist, and change is slow. Insurers often seem to prioritize profits over patient care, frequently issuing denials of care and waiting for someone to dispute them.

In the best of circumstances, filing, refiling, appealing, documenting, tracking, and following up on eating disorder-related insurance claims can take more time, attention, and energy than most people can spare. Doing so while also managing a life-threatening eating disorder is harder, and it's easy to see why insurance denials could lead an individual to think they aren't deserving of care or "sick enough" to need it.

Advocacy organizations, including The International Federation of Eating Disorder Dietitians, The Access to Care Project, The Eating Disorders Coalition, and The Academy of Nutrition and Dietetics, continue to work toward improved insurance coverage for eating disorder care.[8]

References

1. Mahr F, Farahmand P, Bixler EO, et al. A national survey of eating disorder training. *Int J Eat Disord*. 2015;48(4):443-445. doi:10.1002/eat.22335
2. Anderson K, Accurso EC, Kinasz KR, Le Grange D. Residents' and fellows' knowledge and attitudes about eating disorders at an academic medical center. *Acad Psychiatry*. 2017;41(3):381-384. doi:10.1007/s40596-016-0578-z
3. Setnick J, Meseck K, Tackett J, Quatromoni PA. A survey of registered dietitian nutritionists who provide care to clients with eating disorders: implications for education, training, and clinical practice. *J Critical Dietetics*. 2022;6(2):76-90.
4. Kellogg M. When and how to refer to psychotherapy. *Weight Management Matters*. 2008;6(2):14-15.
5. Yager J, Devlin MJ, Halmi KA, et al. *Practice Guideline for The Treatment of Patients With Eating Disorders*. 3rd ed. American Psychiatric Association; 2010. Accessed April 2, 2024. https://psychiatryonline.org/pb/assets/raw/sitewide/practice_guidelines/guidelines/eatingdisorders.pdf
6. Centers for Medicare & Medicaid Services. The Mental Health Parity and Addiction Equity Act (MHPAEA). CMS.gov. 2008. Accessed July 3, 2024. www.cms.gov/marketplace/private-health-insurance/mental-health-parity-addiction-equity
7. Department of the Treasury. Requirements Related to the Mental Health Parity and Addiction Equity Act. Federal Register. 2024. Accessed October 19, 2024. https://www.govinfo.gov/content/pkg/FR-2024-09-23/pdf/2024-20612.pdf
8. International Federation of Eating Disorder Dietitians. IFEDD advocacy initiatives. Accessed October 19, 2024. https://ifedd.org/mhpaea

APPENDIX A

Nutrition Care Process Summary

The Nutrition Care Process (NCP) was designed to clarify and standardize the process that many dietitians perform intuitively. It is represented graphically in Figure A.1 on page 170.

FIGURE A.1 Nutrition Care Process Model

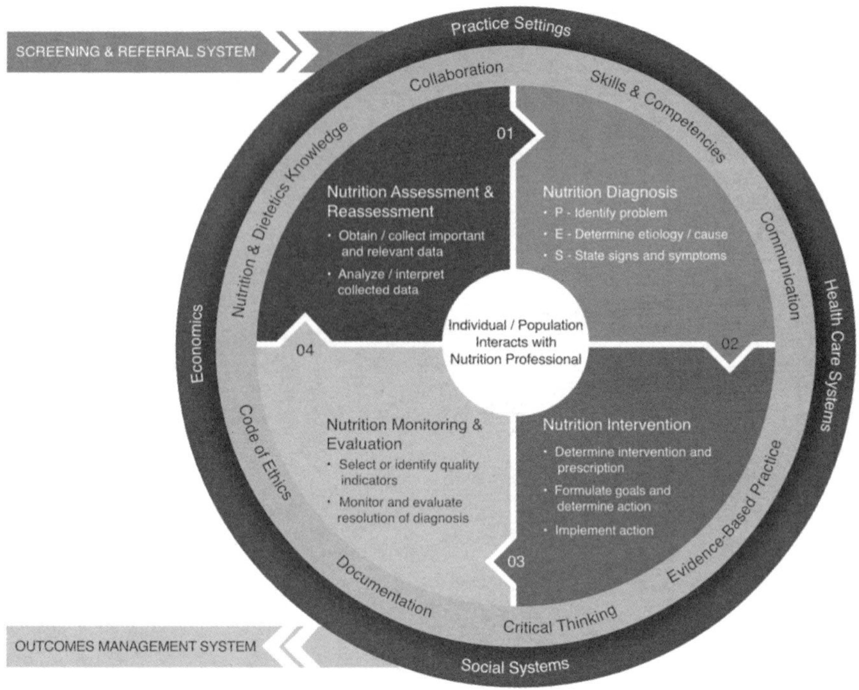

Steps in the Nutrition Care Process

Step 1: Nutrition Assessment

Obtain, verify, and interpret data needed to identify nutrition-related problems, their causes, and significance. Organized into nine domains:

- Food/Nutrition-Related History
- Anthropometric Measurements
- Biochemical Data, Medical Tests, and Procedures
- Physical Exam Findings
- Client History
- Assessment, Monitoring, and Evaluation Tools
- Etiology Category
- Comparative Standards
- Progress Evaluation

Step 2: Nutrition Diagnosis

Identify and describe a specific nutrition problem that can be resolved or improved through treatment/nutrition intervention by a food and nutrition professional. The nutrition diagnosis is conveyed in a problem, etiology, signs and symptoms (PES) statement.

Organized into four domains:

- Intake
- Clinical
- Behavioral-Environmental
- Nutrition Situation

Step 3: Nutrition Intervention

Resolve or improve the nutrition diagnosis or nutrition problem by provision of advice, education, or delivery of the food component of a specific diet or meal plan tailored to the patient's need. The interventions are directed at the etiology of the diagnosis (PES statement). Organized into eight domains:

- Goal planning
- Prescription Planning
- Food and/or Nutrient Delivery
- Nutrition Education
- Nutrition Counseling
- Coordination of Nutrition Care
- Population-Based Nutrition Action
- Nutrition Intervention Encounter Context

Step 4: Nutrition Monitoring and Evaluation

Determine and measure the amount of progress made for the nutrition intervention and whether the nutrition-related goals/outcomes are being met, thus, determining the effectiveness of the interventions by selecting care indicators and the criteria to which the indicator is compared. Organized into eight domains:

- Food/Nutrition-Related History Outcomes
- Anthropometric Measurement Outcomes
- Biochemical Data, Medical Tests, and Procedure Outcomes
- Nutrition Focused Physical Finding Outcomes
- Assessment, Monitoring, and Evaluation Tools
- Etiology Category
- Comparative Standards
- Progress Evaluation

Resource

1. Academy of Nutrition and Dietetics. *Nutrition Care Process Introduction*. 2023. Accessed April 2, 2024. www.ncpro.org/pubs/2023-encpt-en/

APPENDIX B

Guide to Dietary Restrictions

Restrictive eating is not synonymous with dysfunction. There are many reasons for dietary restrictions that are functional and supportive. But religious practice, family tradition, medical necessity, digestive distress, environmental concerns, taste preference, and other aspects can get mixed up with desperation to lose weight prompted by diet culture; fears, anxieties, and traumatic past experiences about eating; and fantasies that eating a certain way will cure a terminal illness or prevent aging. A patient's motivation for dietary restriction may be just as important to evaluate as their eating pattern. Individuals may follow eating rules without knowing if they stem from a personal preference or as an aspect of their eating disorder; it takes time to know the difference.

Box B.1 on page 174 provides the standard guidelines for some common dietary restrictions. Adherence to these guidelines can vary, so before establishing a meal plan, ask each patient about their specific practices.

Expert Insight

A person's personal preferences should be treated with respect as much as possible. If it is in the patient's best interest nutritionally or medically to eat their less-preferred or restricted foods, this should be discussed with the patient directly. Some eating restrictions, including those founded on religious beliefs, allow latitude in light of medical needs. For example, a member of the Muslim faith is allowed to eat nonhalal food if no halal food is available; a member of the Jewish faith is not allowed to fast on even the most holy of fast days if it will harm their health. Patients who are struggling with religious beliefs that conflict with their need for eating disorder treatment may benefit from referral to a religious leader of their faith.

BOX B.1 Explanation of Dietary Restrictions

Name	*Excludes*	*Includes*	*Rationale*
Religious and cultural practices			
Kosher (also called "Kashrus" or "Kashrut"	Pork and all pork products (includes pork gelatin) Shellfish Any one meal may not contain both a dairy product and a meat product Beef and poultry not slaughtered in an approved manner	All grains, fruits, and vegetables Dairy products Fish Beef and poultry certified "Kosher" (K or U inside a circle) Packaged food certified "Kosher"	Jewish religious belief prescribed in the Torah (Old Testament) and practiced by some individuals of the Jewish faith Note: Practices vary widely—assess on an individual basis

BOX B.1 Explanation of Dietary Restrictions (cont.)

Name	*Excludes*	*Includes*	*Rationale*
Halal	Pork and all pork products (includes pork gelatin) Alcohol in any form Beef and poultry not slaughtered in an approved manner	All fruits and vegetables Dairy products Fish Beef and poultry certified "Halal"	Islamic religious belief prescribed in the Quran practiced by some individuals of the Muslim faith Note: Practices vary widely—assess on an individual basis
Lent (Christian Orthodox)	No animal foods are allowed from Ash Wednesday through Easter, except on Sundays	Vegetarian diet daily Unrestricted diet on Sundays	Christian religious belief practiced by members of certain Christian Orthodox faiths Note: Practices vary widely—assess on an individual basis
Lent (Roman Catholic)	Meat from hooved animals (beef and pork) not allowed on Fridays from Ash Wednesday through Easter	Unrestricted diet daily Fish and dairy allowed on Fridays	Christian religious belief practiced by members of the Roman Catholic faith
Lent (Protestant)	Each individual chooses something to "give up for Lent," the period from Ash Wednesday through Easter	The restricted item can be a nonfood item or activity.	Christian religious belief practiced by members of certain Protestant faiths Note: Practices vary widely—assess on an individual basis

Continued on next page

BOX B.1 Explanation of Dietary Restrictions (cont.)

Name	*Excludes*	*Includes*	*Rationale*
Hinduism	Dietary practices vary widely and may include vegetarianism; avoiding meat, fish, and eggs; or just avoidance of beef and beef products	"Sattvic" foods such as fruits, vegetables, nuts, dairy, and grains are considered pure, clean, and beneficial for physical and mental wellness	Hindu religious belief practiced by members of the Hindu faith Note: Practices vary widely—assess on an individual basis
Seventh-day Adventist	No restrictions are required but animal products and alcohol may be avoided by some individuals.	Dietary restrictions are not required but emphasize fruits, vegetables, whole grains, nuts, and legumes	Seventh-day Adventist is a Christian denomination that includes a focus on wellness and healthful living
Plant-based diets			
Semi-vegetarian	All beef, pork, and related products	Poultry Eggs Seafood Dairy	Varies by individual
Pesco-vegetarian	Beef, pork, poultry, and their products	Seafood Dairy Eggs	Varies by individual
Lacto-ovo vegetarian	Beef, pork, poultry, and their products Seafood	Dairy Eggs	Varies by individual
Lacto-vegetarian	Beef, pork, poultry, and their products Seafood Eggs	Dairy	Varies by individual

BOX B.1 Explanation of Dietary Restrictions (cont.)

Name	*Excludes*	*Includes*	*Rationale*
Vegan	All animal products	All plant foods	Varies by individual
Raw foods	Cooked food Processed food Food heated to > 116 °F	Vegetables Fruits (fresh or dried) Sprouts Nuts and seeds Grains Beans Seaweed	Belief that heating food destroys digestive enzymes and that cooking diminishes the nutritional value and "life-force" of food
Macrobiotic	All animal products Certain fruits and juice Coffee Processed foods Artificial ingredients	Beans Vegetables Tofu Whole grains Tea	Live "in balance with nature" for a healthy mind, body, and spirit
Medical diets			
Low FODMAP	Foods low in FODMAPs: Some fruits and vegetables, rice, oats, quinoa, corn, buckwheat, millet Lactose-free dairy Most meats and poultry, fish, seafood, eggs Most fats and oils	Wheat, onions, garlic, legumes, dairy products, honey, high-fructose corn syrup, sugar alcohols	Elimination diet intended to be implemented for 2 to 6 weeks, after which foods are reintroduced to determine which cause digestive symptoms

Continued on next page

Guide to Dietary Restrictions

BOX B.1 Explanation of Dietary Restrictions (cont.)

Name	***Excludes***	***Includes***	***Rationale***
Gluten-free	Wheat, rye, barley, and all foods containing them, their flour, or their gluten storage proteins: gliadin, secalin, and hordein Most baked goods, pastas, and cereals Processed foods with gluten-related ingredients	All meats Fish Poultry Eggs Corn, quinoa, rice Legumes Nuts and seeds Dairy Fruits Vegetables Baked goods and pasta made from gluten-free flours	Medical diet for celiac disease or gluten intolerance Note: Following a gluten-free diet prior to diagnosis of celiac disease can confound test results and cause a false-negative reading
Ketogenic	Limits carbohydrate intake from all sources to 20 to 40 g/d	Heavy cream, full-fat cheese and butter, leafy greens, fish, meat, poultry, eggs	Used to prevent seizures
Other			
Calorie restriction	Processed sugars Flour "Calorie-sparse" foods Red meat White rice	Vegetables Small amounts of fish Nutrition supplements	Based on rats who lived longer in studies when placed on a calorie-restricted diet

BOX B.1 Explanation of Dietary Restrictions (cont.)

Name	*Excludes*	*Includes*	*Rationale*
Paleo	Cereal grains, legumes (including peanuts) Dairy Refined sugar Potatoes Processed foods Refined vegetable oils	Grass-fed meats Fish and seafood Fresh fruits Vegetables Eggs Nuts and seeds Olive, walnut, flaxseed, macadamia, avocado, and coconut oils	A diet that our distant ancestors ate before the advent of agriculture
Keto	Fruit (except berries) Grains Starchy vegetables and "high-sugar" fruits Sweetened yogurt Juices Honey, syrup, or sugar in any form Chips and crackers Baked goods including gluten-free baked goods	Fish, seafood, poultry Eggs "Low-carb" vegetables Cheese, butter, cream, sour cream, Greek yogurt, cottage cheese Avocados Berries Nuts and seeds Olive oil	Health or weight loss

Abbreviation: FODMAP, fermentable oligosaccharides, disaccharides, monosaccharides, and polyols.

APPENDIX C

Caffeine Content in Common Foods, Beverages, and Drugs

	Serving size	Caffeine (mg)
Caffeine drinks[a]		
5-Hour Energy Extra Strength	1.9 fl oz	230
5-Hour Energy Regular Strength	1.5 fl oz	200
7Up, Fanta, Fresca, ginger ale, Sprite	12 fl oz	0
AHA+ Coffee Sparkling Water	12 fl oz	30
AHA+ Green Tea Sparkling Water	12 fl oz	30
AMP Energy Boost Original (PepsiCo)	16 fl oz	142
Arizona Iced Tea, green, all varieties	16 fl oz	15
Bai Antioxidant Infusion	18 fl oz	55
Barq's Root Beer, regular	12 fl oz	23
Bubly Bounce Caffeinated Sparkling Water	12 fl oz	35
Coca-Cola Life	12 fl oz 20 fl oz	27 45
Coca-Cola, Coke Zero, or Diet Pepsi	12 fl oz 20 fl oz	35 58
Diet Coke	12 fl oz 20 fl oz	47 78

Caffeine Content in Common Foods, Beverages, and Drugs (cont.)		
	Serving size	**Caffeine (mg)**
Caffeine drinks[a] (cont.)		
Dr Pepper or Sunkist, regular or diet	12 fl oz 20 fl oz	41 68
Full Throttle (Monster)	16 fl oz	200
Glacéau Vitaminwater Energy	20 fl oz	50
Lipton 100% Natural Lemon Iced Tea, bottle	20 fl oz	35
Lipton Decaffeinated Tea—black or green, brewed	8 fl oz	5
Lipton Pure Leaf Iced Tea	18.5 fl oz	60
Monster Energy	16 fl oz	160
Mountain Dew Kick Start	16 fl oz	92
Mountain Dew, regular or diet	12 fl oz 20 fl oz	54 90
Mountain Zevia (Zevia)	12 fl oz	55
NOS Energy Drink (Monster)	16 fl oz	160
Ocean Spray Cran-Energy	20 fl oz	55
Panera Charged Lemonade	20 fl oz	156
Panera Charged Splash	20 fl oz	124
Pepsi	12 fl oz 20 fl oz	38 63
Pepsi MAX	12 fl oz	69
Pepsi True	7.5 fl oz 20 fl oz	24 64
Phocus Sparkling Water	11.5 fl oz	75
Rockstar	16 fl oz	160
Rockstar Citrus Punched	16 fl oz	240
Root beer, most brands, or Barq's Diet Root Beer	12 fl oz	0

Continued on next page

Caffeine Content in Common Foods, Beverages, and Drugs (cont.)		
	Serving size	**Caffeine (mg)**
Caffeine drinks[a] (cont.)		
Silk chocolate soy milk	8 fl oz	4
Starbucks Caffè Mocha	6 fl oz	175
Starbucks Coffee	12 fl oz	260
Starbucks Coffee	16 fl oz	330
Starbucks Coffee	20 fl oz	415
Starbucks Chai Latte—hot or iced	16 fl oz	95
Starbucks Doubleshot Energy Coffee, can	15 fl oz	146
Starbucks Espresso	doppio (2 oz)	150
Starbucks Espresso Frappuccino	24 fl oz	185
Starbucks Frappuccino Coffee, bottle	9.5 fl oz	90
Starbucks Hot Chocolate	16 fl oz	25
Starbucks Iced Coffee	6 fl oz	165
Starbucks Refreshers	12 fl oz	50
Starbucks Tazo Awake—Brewed Tea or Tea Latte	16 fl oz	135
Starbucks Tazo Chai Tea Latte	16 fl oz	95
Starbucks Tazo Earl Grey Brewed Tea or Tea Latte	16 fl oz	115
Starbucks Tripleshot Energy	8 fl oz	35
Surge	20 fl oz	87
V8 V-Fusion+Energy	8 fl oz	80
Venom Energy Drink (Dr Pepper/Seven Up Inc)	16 fl oz	160
Water Joe	20 fl oz	70

Caffeine Content in Common Foods, Beverages, and Drugs (cont.)	Serving size	Caffeine (mg)
Frozen desserts		
Bang!! Caffeinated Ice Cream	4 fl oz	125
Baskin Robbins Jamoca Ice Cream	4 fl oz	20
Ben & Jerry's Coffee Ice Cream	2/3 cup	47
Breyers Coffee Ice Cream	4 fl oz	1
Cold Stone Creamery Mocha Ice Cream	12 fl oz	52
Dannon All Natural Coffee Low-Fat Yogurt	6 oz	30
Dreyer's or Edy's Grand Ice Cream—Coffee or Espresso Chip	4 fl oz	17
Dreyer's, Edy's, or Häagen-Dazs Chocolate Ice Cream	4 fl oz	less than 1
Häagen-Dazs Coffee Almond Crunch Snack Size Bar	1.8 oz	10
Häagen-Dazs Coffee Ice Cream	4 fl oz	29
Starbucks Coffee Ice Cream	4 fl oz	45
Starbucks Mocha Frappuccino Ice Cream	4 fl oz	25
Stonyfield Gotta Have Java Nonfat Frozen Yogurt	4 fl oz	28
TCBY Coffee Frozen Yogurt	13.4 fl oz	42
Chocolates/candies/other		
Awake Caffeinated Chocolate Bar	1.55 oz	101
Awake Caffeinated Chocolate Bites	0.53 oz	50
Blue Diamond Almonds, Roasted Coffee Flavored	1 oz	25
Clif Shot Energy Gel	1 packet	100

Continued on next page

Caffeine Content in Common Foods, Beverages, and Drugs (cont.)		
	Serving size	**Caffeine (mg)**
Chocolates/candies/other (cont.)		
Crackheads	1 box, 40 g	600
Crackheads Espresso Bean Candies, regular	1 package (28 pieces)	200
Crystal Light Energy	½ packet	60
Dove Dark Chocolate Silky Smooth Promises	5 pieces	4
G endurance energy gel	1 packet	30
Gu energy gel	1 packet	20-40
Gu energy stroop waffle	1.1 oz waffle	20
Hershey's Cocoa	1 Tbsp	8
Hershey's Kisses	9 pieces	9
Hershey's Special Dark Chocolate Bar	1.5 oz	20
Hershey's—Milk Chocolate Bar	1.6 oz	9
Hydrant	0.3 oz packet	100
Jelly Belly Extreme Sport Beans	1 package	50
Jolt Gum	1 piece	45
MiO Energy, all flavors	1 squirt, ½ tsp	60
Muscle Milk Orange Energy Chews	1.27 oz	30
Nuun Sport + Caffeine	1 tablet; 16 oz	40
Perky Jerky	1 oz	10
Run Gum Extra Strength	1 piece	100
Run Gum Energy Gum	1 piece	50
Skratch Labs Sport Energy Chews	1.8 oz	50
Wired Waffles	1 waffle	200

Caffeine Content in Common Foods, Beverages, and Drugs (cont.)	Serving size	Caffeine (mg)
Over-the-counter drugs		
Anacin	2 tablets	64
Bayer Back & Body	2 caplets	65
Excedrin Migraine	2 tablets	130
Jet-Alert regular strength	1 tablet	100
Midol Complete	2 caplets	120
NoDoz or Vivarin	1 caplet	200
Zantrex-3 weight-loss supplement	2 capsules	300

[a] The US Food and Drug Administration sets the limit for cola and pepper soft drinks at 71 mg (200 parts per million) per 12 oz serving.

Sources: Center for Science in the Public Interest. Caffeine chart. Updated 2020-2024. Accessed January 2024. www.cspinet.org/caffeine-chart

Additional information: Juliano LM, Griffiths RR. Caffeine. In: Lowinson JH, Ruiz P, Millman RB, Langrod JG, eds. *Substance Abuse: A Comprehensive Textbook*. 4th ed. Lippincott, Williams & Wilkins; 2005:403-421.

APPENDIX D

Additional Resources

Books Written by Dietitians

Anti-Diet: Reclaim Your Time, Money, Well-Being, and Happiness Through Intuitive Eating, by Christy Harrison

Beat Body Bullying and Learn to Love Yourself, by Jessika Brown

Body Kindness: Transform Your Health from the Inside Out—and Never Say Diet Again, by Rebecca Scritchfield

Born To Eat: Whole, Healthy Foods from Baby's First Bite, by Leslie Schilling and Wendy Jo Peterson

Counseling Tips for Nutrition Therapists: Practice Workbook Series, by Molly Kellogg

Eat to Love, by Jenna Hollenstein

The Eating Disorder Clinical Pocket Guide: Quick Reference for Healthcare Providers, by Jessica Setnick

The Eating Disorder Trap: A Guide for Clinicians and Loved Ones, by Robyn Goldberg

Feed Yourself: Step Away from the Lies of Diet Culture and Into Your Divine Design, by Leslie Schilling

How to Nourish Your Child Through an Eating Disorder: A Simple, Plate-By-Plate Approach to Rebuilding a Healthy Relationship With Food, by Casey Crosbie and Wendy Sterling

Intuitive Eating: A Revolutionary Anti-Diet Approach, 4th edition, by Evelyn Tribole and Elyse Resch and *The Intuitive Eating Workbook: Ten Principles for Nourishing a Healthy Relationship With Food*

Intuitive Eating for Life, by Jenna Hollenstein

It's Always Been Ours: Rewriting the Story of Black Women's Bodies, by Jessica Wilson

Love Your Body: Change the Way You Feel About the Body You Have, by Tami Brannon-Quan and Lisa Licavoli

Moving Away from Diets: Healing Eating Problems and Exercise Resistance, 2nd edition, by Karin Kratina, Nancy King, and Dayle Hayes

Nancy Clark's Sports Nutrition Guidebook, 5th edition, by Nancy Clark

Nourish: How to Heal Your Relationship With Food, Body and Self, by Heidi Schauster

No Weigh! A Teen's Guide to Positive Body Image, Food, and Emotional Wisdom, by Wendy Sterling, Signe Darpinian, and Shelley Aggarwal

Nutrition Counseling and Communication Skills, by Katharine Curry and Amy Jaffe

Nutrition Counseling in the Treatment of Eating Disorders, 2nd edition, by Marcia Herrin and Maria Larkin

PCOS: The Dietitian's Guide, 2nd edition, by Angela Grassi

Recover: Finding Freedom With Food Again, by Sunny Yingling

Unworthy Weight: Reclaiming Your Worth from a Number on a Scale and Finding True Identity in Christ, by Kristin Williams

Winning the War Within: Nutrition Therapy for Clients With Eating Disorders, 3rd edition, by Eileen Stellefson Myers and Charlotte Caperton-Kilburn

Continuing Professional Education and Additional Notes

This edition of *Academy of Nutrition and Dietetics Pocket Guide to Eating Disorders* offers readers Continuing Professional Education (CPE) credit. Please check the expiration date and the number of hours offered at the link that follows or on the product page at www.eatrightSTORE.org. Readers may earn credit by completing the interactive online quiz at: https://publications.webauthor.com/PG_ED_3e

The Academy of Nutrition and Dietetics Product Strategy & Revenue Operations team can be reached at publications@eatright.org. Additional notes, errata, related products, and information on licensing and permissions can be found on the product page at www.eatrightSTORE.org or at the QR code below.

Index

Letters *b*, *f*, and *t* after page number indicate box, figure, and table, respectively.